Kat Brown is a freelance journalist and commentator whose work, covering arts and entertainment as well as her experience with infertility and adult ADHD diagnosis, has appeared across national print and broadcast. She has published two books within one month of each other (which is very ADHD), *No One Talks About This Stuff* (ed.) and *It's Not A Bloody Trend: Understanding Life as an ADHD Adult*. She loves horse riding, tarot and quizzes, and captained The Jillies on BBC Two's *Only Connect* – arguably the greatest quiz show in existence. Kat lives in South London with her husband, their dog, and two appalling cats.

'Raw, honest and open . . . Kat could not have described *No One Talks About This Stuff* more perfectly by saying it is a support group in a book; it is that, and so much more'

Pippa Vosper, author of *Beyond Grief*

'Shining a warm light on the stories that should never have sat in the shadows . . . This book welcomes knowing nods, valuable insight, and hope to those who are tired of sitting behind the taboo. Life affirming, searingly honest and deeply moving'

Anna Mathur, author of *Know Your Worth*

'Kat Brown's constellation of stories explores the persistently misunderstood experience of reproductive loss. The voices of the contributors are necessarily varied, but they are unified by fascinating and moving insights'

Julia Bueno, author of *The Brink of Being*

# NO ONE TALKS ABOUT THIS STUFF

### TWENTY-TWO STORIES OF ALMOST PARENTHOOD

### EDITED BY KAT BROWN

unbound

First published in 2024

Unbound
c/o TC Group, 6th Floor King's House, 9–10 Haymarket, London SW1Y 4BP
www.unbound.com

Typeset by Jouve (UK), Milton Keynes

A CIP record for this book is available from the British Library

ISBN 978-1-80018-287-5 (paperback)
ISBN 978-1-80018-288-2 (ebook)

Printed in Great Britain by Clays Ltd, Elcograf S.p.A.

1 3 5 7 9 8 6 4 2

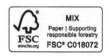

MIX
Paper | Supporting
responsible forestry
FSC® C018072

For Will, Matt and Wheats, who believed in me and this book when they absolutely did not have to.

And for my darling Harry for everything, always.

## Editor's Note

For years, my main cultural touchstone with infertility was the author Jilly Cooper, who wrote her own experience of recurrent miscarriage and adoption into her heroes Rupert and Taggie Campbell-Black. Cheers to you, Jilly, and thank you for all you have done to make infertility a blockbuster plot point rather than a hidden one. I hope Disney paid you an absolute fortune for *Rivals*.

# Contents

# Introduction

This is the book that I wish I'd found in the bookshops when my husband and I were trying for a baby. The infertility bookshelf felt very small then, often tucked in beside parenting and 'miracle-baby' memoirs, as though the unthinkable never happened to anyone, and if it did, it ended with a nursery-makeover Pinterest board and a lovely rainbow. For a few years we tried 'naturally' (ovulation sticks, diaries and apps – so natural), then moved on to examinations, operations and treatment. It never occurred to me that our journey to having children would end after two IVF cycles. As I understood it, if we kept putting tokens in the slot machine, we would eventually have a baby.

After our treatment failed, I fell apart like a box of Shredded Wheat dropped from a great height. My husband found me a new therapist who specialised in infertility. She looked about twenty, and we called her TCT: Terrifyingly Competent Therapist. I respected and admired her, and she helped me to heal until I ghosted her the following winter. She thoughtfully suggested that we might hold a funeral for our unborn children to honour them.

I said this was a wonderful idea, and then I never spoke to her again.

I couldn't hold a funeral because how could it just be us two who loved our children? How could I ask our friends and family to come to a funeral where the only things being buried were memories of people who were real to us yet didn't exist? How could I equate this thin misery to the lovely christenings, weddings and birthdays we celebrated? How could I subject them to this? And, in a much smaller voice, I thought: *How could I dare to ask them to hold me through it?*

In therapy, I'd written a great long letter to my children. I'd even imagined them sitting in the armchair as I talked to them, but I wasn't ready to say goodbye. In the early spring, my husband and I made an appointment with a new IVF clinic, where we planned to try an 'all you can eat' option where you fork over a lot of money and then keep . . . having . . . IVF until you have a child or go insane. I had been ill with a shopping list of mental health problems for many years, so I was pretty confident I could cope. We had been given three cycles of IVF on the NHS, but as none of my eggs had been mature enough to fertilise on our first cycle, that was the end of that. We paid for the next one ourselves – the same outcome. Now we could keep paying.

Our appointment at this second clinic was cancelled because our consultant, in an unfortunate pastiche of private doctors, had broken their leg skiing. By the time we rescheduled, we had gone into lockdown, which is why my husband and I were hunched over my iPhone on speaker mode as the consultant told us that they couldn't, in all good faith, recommend we do any further IVF. It wasn't going to work for us. There would be no pass Go, collect a baby, and forget. We walked out of the house and under the grey-nothing March skies, walking in silence to Brockwell Park and then home again.

I had been so confident that IVF would work, partly because I have the unquestioning optimism of a golden retriever and partly because the science didn't show any reason for it not to. My AMH levels were excellent, at thirty-five I was young (ish), and at the grim heart of it I knew that the world was filled with women becoming pregnant during the darkest times. 'Stress' wasn't going to prevent me from getting knocked up.

When I found out that treatment had again not worked due to my eggs not maturing, it was as though I had entered a black hole of grief. I left all my WhatsApp groups and sent a public tweet to comprehensively cover any well-wishers and make it clear that I just wanted comfort: 'I've just found out that our second round of IVF hasn't worked, for reasons that mean that I will probably never be able to have a baby. If you have time to send good thoughts, I would really appreciate it. I never knew I could feel so ill or so sad.'

Was this an appropriate reaction? I don't know. There aren't books about what to do in these situations. Etiquette guides have no advice on how to word a notice in *The Times* that you are welcoming a little bundle of nothing. I shouted my grief into the world, begging that someone anonymous would hear me and carry it for me so that I didn't have to ask friends or family, because I didn't trust that they wouldn't leave me to it. I judged them all so unfairly because that was how I saw myself. I didn't know anyone who had tried IVF and not had it work, eventually. That was the story: you emerged sad, bruised, broken – and with a child.

There was nowhere I could call: there were charities for infertility, miscarriage, stillbirth or for parents whose children had died. I hadn't miscarried. I hadn't experienced any of these dreadful tragedies, and yet, oh God, I *had* lost a child. I could see my children so clearly. These lives would have been growing with me and my husband. Our little family, quickly becoming a huge family because we're both ridiculously tall. There are so many little stings in infertility that you suck up until suddenly you are queueing in the post office, flayed alive. All the nurseries and school runs I'd looked into from our house, the ridiculous arguments over names we'd had (of all the possibilities in Terry Pratchett's 'Discworld' novels, why 'Havelock'?), the friends we'd chosen to be godparents, the little gingerbread *Star Wars* outfit I'd bought from GAP one Christmas and hidden in a cupboard.

My grief was a rebellious Victorian child who must sit neatly and cleanly in its Sunday best while grown-ups talk about boring things, instead of doing what it wanted to do, which was to run screaming into the garden and up the nearest tree, to feel the sun on its face, to hide away to read for hours, and to make no small talk whatsoever. I lost the ability to be appropriate when well-meaning strangers asked if I had children, or would like children, or any other questions that people feel they can ask women that essentially amount to 'conversations about your vagina'. Someone didn't speak to me for months because my infertility was taking away from their being able to take joy in their pregnancy. I swallowed down everything I could to try and smooth this out and didn't speak to them about it further. I thought I might actually kill them if I did.

But if people were to ask me about my children, what

would I say? That my husband and I never could decide on a name for a boy (apologies to all Havelocks, but no), which means that I would have exercised triumphant veto for reasons of Being The One Who Pushed The Bloody Thing Out. I didn't think of my not-children all the time, but I loved them. I saw them in the corner of my eye like will-o'-the-wisps, these spirits of another timeline in which my husband and I were parents watching these tiny feral pixies gradually unfolding into the people they would become.

If you've written a CV, you'll know that life only makes sense when you can pull it into some semblance of a story, discarding the bits that don't add to it, even though they are all part of the foggy muddle that took you to wherever you are. It's easy to look back and fixate on the moments that didn't happen how you wanted – or at all – and think, *If only I had gone down that path, I would be amazing, incredible, happy.* This book asks: how do we make sense of a world in which we can see another path, but have been unable to take it? Perhaps it feels as though we are living it simultaneously, papered thinly over until the joins are smoothed away, and all that is left is confusion, not living in one reality or the other. I had no clear path to go down when motherhood was cut off to me.

I found comfort of a sort in learning about disenfranchised grief; the term coined by the grief specialist Kenneth Doka in his 1989 book of the same name to describe a loss that isn't acknowledged by wider society: a beloved pet dying, missing out on a celebration because of Covid, or mourning the children you were never pregnant with. I found still more in Kate Bowler's podcast *Everything Happens.* Her plans to expand her family were cut short when she was diagnosed with stage-four colorectal cancer at thirty-five, and in a kind, funny and compassionate way, she interviews people about the times that positive affirmations can't get you through. Listening to people like me, not only celebrities, talking about their darkest moments and how they found the courage to keep going anchored me at a time when I worried that, if I didn't pay close enough attention, I would float away.

For that reason, I am very grateful to the writers who agreed to be part of this book before I even launched it and to the 200 people who answered my call for public submissions so this book could have the broadest possible range of viewpoints and experiences. Talking about 'this stuff' can be hard even when you are a little further down the path, but this response shows the kindness of people who are willing to share their stories with others.

This book is very selfish in that I hoped it would help me just as much as the reader. I have always found reassurance in what others say about life. It helps to hear people share how they deal with their nightmares, how they continue to put one foot in front of the other and do the next right thing. 'Listen for the similarities and not the differences,' as the saying goes in Twelve Step programmes. The details in someone's story might be unfamiliar, but the emotions are entirely known.

Whatever pain might keep you from peace, whatever path your mind keeps trying to go down, I hope that you will find comfort here, and perhaps begin your own conversations. There is common ground to be had when someone tells their story honestly, even more so when it is about something that has been kept in the shadows. Emerge from them. You are seen, you are heard, and you are real.

Kat Brown, Streatham Hill, March 2024

# Disenfranchised Grief

# The Story Which Does Not Have an End

*Alice Jolly*

It is the summer of 1989, and I am leaving university. I should possess a photo of this moment, but I don't. Yet I can imagine how we looked. A group of young women with fluffy hair, shoulder pads, smoky eyeliner, standing in a line, raising our glasses to our brilliant futures. We are the New Generation, daughters of Women's Lib. We take it for granted that we will have houses in London, jobs as lawyers, management consultants, doctors. This is our Age of Innocence, and we never think of what lies ahead.

Now, over thirty years later, we look back on our lives and see the wreckage. Not the major wreckage of climate change, or Covid, or austerity, but simply the small wreckage of average lives. For what no one had told us is that even in an average life there will almost certainly be appalling tragedy. Much of that tragedy arises from the decision to bring children into the world – or not.

In our university days, children were mere wallpaper. They decorated the imagined house in Hampstead or the Cotswolds. The business of actually having children was gross, repulsive. We giggled in the bookshop over the 600-page tome called

*Preparing for Pregnancy* even though some had already discovered how dangerously easy pregnancy can be. The horrors of the abortion clinic purposefully wiped from the mind.

A few years later, when we decided that the time was right to have children, we had no idea that we were entering a cruel and brutal lottery. We had been brought up to believe that we could get what we wanted by trying hard, passing exams, meeting the right people. If you decided to have children, you would have them. It was like buying a car.

Yet all too soon we understood that some women push out three children without a second thought. Others perhaps have a miscarriage or two but that is soon forgotten in the joys of their living children. Then there are the Unfortunates. You hope you won't meet them at a party. What can one say? So sad.

You understand that I am not writing here about an idealised world. Instead, I am writing about what we actually think and feel about fertility and infertility, childbearing, loss. I am writing about our cheap motivations, our bitchy thoughts, our love of scapegoating. What might we say if we decided to be nakedly honest about *the stuff* that *no one talks about?*

When we hear of the failure of our friend's fifth round of IVF or our cousin's third miscarriage – what really passes through our minds? Even as we offer our words of comfort we think, *Thank God I am not her.* Secretly we may also be just a little pleased. We live in a highly competitive world. Babies are a prize. Too often, we do not really sympathise with the loser. Instead, we tell ourselves that our cousin, or our friend, was always a little too pleased with herself.

4

Also, we secretly believe that the miscarriage or the failed IVF was her fault. In order to maintain this narrative, we need to find causes. She married a man who is years older. She is so stressed. She left it too late. She put her job before everything else and this is the result. She is overweight; she is underweight. She gets her hair coloured; she smokes.

Don't tell me you haven't played this game. Whether victim or perpetrator, winner or loser, we have all had these thoughts. But why? Because we are frightened. Very frightened. We hide behind the certainty that we are the wise virgins and have tended our lamps. In ancient societies, people hung herbs outside the door to prevent the devil from entering. These stories of fault are the modern herbs-at-the-door, the talismans which we use to ensure that disaster will pass us by.

My husband and I were among the Unfortunates. When our second child was stillborn, our Age of Innocence came to an abrupt end. In my childhood, I had vaguely heard of still-births. There was the family at the school gate. *That family. The baby. Shocking.* Forced smiles were displayed as the mother walked by. Suddenly I became that woman.

I so badly needed comfort yet instead I spent my time comforting other women. *You mustn't feel bad. Really, I am doing fine.* It was a relief when a friend said, *Whenever I think of you then I just hug my children and feel really, really lucky.* What she was acknowledging is that survivor's guilt is a pointless emotion which burdens both the victim and the person who feels the guilt.

Initially, I simply couldn't navigate the drastically changed world I had come to inhabit. I was frequently left gasping and wounded by the inappropriate things other people said or did. But grief has its rules and eventually I learnt them. Keep it clean and tidy. Do upbeat things. Like raising money for charity or working for a local stillbirth support group. Do not weep copiously at dinner parties. Do not make the people with the living babies feel bad. Do not cause embarrassment. And most importantly, do not be bitter or self-pitying.

Why do we fear the people who are grieving in unacceptable ways? The reality is that none of us want to be too close to people who are repeatedly pointing out how hard and brutal life is, who are reminding us that there is no sense or justice in it. If these facts are made explicit, then the fragile structures which support our lives begin to break apart. We all need hope, but we also need the truth. How do we find a balance between those incompatible needs?

In our case, medical negligence was the talisman of choice for friends and family. My husband is a lawyer, so we live in a world where people put faith in the ability of the law to move disordered events back into the realm of the rational. *You were let down by the hospital and the law must hold the hospital to account. You must fight for justice so that the same thing doesn't happen to others.*

The only problem was that my husband and I did not agree with this version of events. We both felt that the care we had received was good. Our daughter had died in a Belgian hospital and the healthcare system in that country is excellent. I didn't want to fight a legal case so that others could feel better. So much easier to talk about the law than to say, 'We were let down by the nature of this world. And the same could happen to you. Any time, any day.'

*

6

For us, it didn't end there. Things got worse, bigger, more difficult. Recurrent miscarriages, failed IVF, plans to adopt which misfired. Who knew that babies were so unevenly distributed? There comes a moment when even your good friends leave you bleeding on the side of the road. I say this without accusation or blame. I also wanted to leave me on the side of the road. An irreparable hole was blown in just about every friendship we'd ever had.

*Thank God it wasn't me.* Is that what people were saying, or thinking? Yes and no. There is also the desire to be part of the drama. To be the centre of attention. There comes a moment when the story becomes so big that people write newspaper articles and everyone wants a part of it. I finished up writing a memoir because I was bored with other people telling my story inaccurately.

But it turned out that my actual story was not wanted. No one was interested in publishing the memoir I wrote. A story needs to be the right size to be told. Big but not too big. Our story was too big and I was not telling it in a nice way. It was all too sad and *people don't really want to know about difficult women's stuff.*

But Unbound did publish the book (thank you so much!). And that book was followed by a flood of other memoirs focused on women's relationships with their own bodies. I am not boastful enough to think that I made that possible. But it is important to remember that a taboo is not something no one wants to talk about. It is something everyone wants to talk about but no one knows where to start. This current anthology is another way of opening the conversation about *this stuff.*

*

So, are times changing? Are we now more open, more compassionate in the way we speak about fertility and infertility, loss and childlessness? Yes, but not always in ways that are positive. I teach life writing and I have seen the way in which writing personal stories has become an industry. Personal pain is treated as a commodity, a part of the Great Competition. *Oh, you think to impress me with your four miscarriages. Lay out your dead babies and let me see if they are as good as mine.*

We operate in a world where being a victim is a mark of status. If you do not have your own pain, then you requisition the pain of others. If you do not have a bad-news story to tell, then you are not a real person and your right to speak is in question. We want to avoid pain, to deny it, to push it aside. But to be in pain is also to be alive and, in a world where we are increasingly disengaged from our own lives, pain is the opportunity to touch something real.

I hate being the person who plays the trump card, who wins the Pain Olympics. A stillbirth, four miscarriages, failed IVF, stalled attempts to adopt. I also hate being the person who is so brave because look how she has carried on, remade her life. (Subtext: you lesser Unfortunates should stop feeling so sorry for yourselves.)

I wish that we could be in control of the way in which our stories are received and processed, but we cannot. We have to accept that when we speak the truth, we will soon find it twisted. We have to be honest about the ways in which that happens, and we have to acknowledge the part that we ourselves sometimes play in that process. We need to recognise the unpleasantly competitive nature of our late-stage-capitalism world, the bitchiness, the lost friendships, the blame. But then we have to lay all that aside and remember that, in reality, there is no community so close as the one welded together by grief that is openly and honestly expressed.

I personally do not consider myself a victim. I consider myself lucky, spectacularly lucky. I finished up with three children. One dead but still alive in our hearts. The third born through surrogacy and egg donation. That decision to use a surrogate mum in America and also an egg donor was massive, extreme. The birth of our daughter in a distant corner of Minnesota still feels like some strange dream.

Of course, before we made our choices, we worried about whether it would matter that our daughter (whom we named Hope) is not genetically related to me. Just for the record, it never has. Not for one moment. But what of our daughter? Does it matter to her? For the moment, it does not. She is also a child of a New Generation and, even as a four-year-old, she took the measure of the competitive nature of the world and decided to win. She has a Whopping Story to tell, and she is going to tell it to anyone who will listen (plus those who have failed to edge out of the room fast enough).

At the school nativity she told the whole audience that although Baby Jesus was born in Bethlehem, she herself was born in America. *No way is that Baby Jesus going to get one up on me.* More recently, as I am doing a chicken walk around the kitchen (as you do), Hope sighs and rolls her eyes, says, 'Thank God I am not related to you.'

I remind her that we may not be genetically related, but I am her mother.

More sighing and eye rolling. *Don't you understand about genes?* She starts to give me chapter and verse on genes as

I hurriedly back out of the room. I am just grateful for her scientific mind and a new age in which questions of 'blood' are not dark and shameful in the way that they once were.

Of course, Hope is only ten. Doubtless the teenage years will be more difficult, but then they always are, no matter the nature of the family. Just yesterday she came home from school and said that a girl at school keeps saying 'Hope is adopted'. This continues even though Hope has explained *everything* about genes. Is that upsetting? I ask. No, just boring. Really boring.

I also feel lucky because at least things happened to us. People were interested in the soap opera of our struggles – even if their interest was largely just shock-horror, ring-all-your-friends-and-gasp. Worse is the people for whom nothing happens. Nothing at all. They just never get pregnant. A miscarriage is bad, but it is the chance of a living baby. For people who never get pregnant, there is nothing to see, nothing to grieve. People make an assumption that they never wanted children.

Where does this leave us? What was the point that I wanted to make? Thirty-five years have passed since that non-existent university leaving photo, our brief Age of Innocence. My stillborn daughter Laura would now be seventeen. Those women of my youth are kinder now. That's another thing they don't tell you. People generally do get kinder as they get older. All that competitiveness and ambition and jealousy drop away.

My understanding of what happened to us has also changed. There are plenty of friendships that were never mended and never will mend. I can still finish up in a bitter rage about tactless things that were said and done. But I do also forgive. I acknowledge that I too have failed many people and said, or done, the wrong thing.

Even now I sometimes receive emails and calls from former colleagues, or the daughters of friends, who are going through infertility issues and want to talk. Sometimes I send a polite but firmly negative one-line email. Sometimes I do not respond at all. I am not proud of that. But I know now that there are moments when we can offer sympathy, kindness, tea and chats. And other moments when we cannot offer anything much at all.

We all have to recognise that we cannot be friends to everyone. I can forgive myself now for my moments of failure and also for some of the things that I said and did during those gruelling and painful years. I am not an easy person to help. I was brought up to be a woman who gives, not a woman who receives. I froze people out. I did not know then that you have to take what people are offering and be grateful – even when it is not what you need or want.

I couldn't help myself at that time and so, inevitably, I didn't know how to ask others for what I wanted. Anyway, what I really wanted – to bring our daughter back from the dead – was totally impossible. That itself was a part of the anger. So much to forgive. Also, now the growing realisation that forgiveness is not a moment in time. It is something you have to do every day. It is an ongoing project, it is hard work, it has no end.

My generation are mainly just glad to find themselves still here. What I saw in my thirties, others are only seeing now.

Your fifties are like snipers' alley. Some are not going to make it through. Occasionally, people say to me now that they feel they are suddenly beginning to understand what it might have felt like for us. I have no desire to say, 'I told you so'.

I am just sorry that they have to know, that we all have to know sometime. I am in danger of becoming that older woman who says, 'This too will pass.' True, it will pass, but that is of no help when you are in the middle of it. It will pass but you will also be dead. Is that better? Yes, you can try to find a nice way to tell the story. You can learn some useful lessons. You can raise money for charity. You can campaign for better medical care for women.

All these things are certainly worth doing. We can all learn to find ways to turn our losses into something positive. We can all laugh in the lifeboats. You may have days when you think that you just cannot carry on for one moment more. But the bitter truth is that the days keep coming whether you want them or not. Unless you can find the organisational skills necessary for gas or ropes or razors.

But what I would really like to do is to sit beside you and put my arm around you and let you talk endlessly – on and on and on – in a messy and angry and bitter and self-pitying way. I want to hear your story. I want to make a space where you can say that it is desperately hard, that it hurts like hell. And it is abysmally unfair and there is no sense in it.

You are not at fault. Your partner is not at fault. You do not have to learn lessons and become a better person. It is not true that what doesn't kill you makes you stronger. Pain can make you small and bitter and nasty. Let us just say, let us just be honest – all this is just bad luck. Bad, bad luck. Nothing can compensate for losses of this kind. Nothing. Weep messily at the bottom of the bed whenever you feel the need. Say bitter things to blameless people. Rage against the world and how appallingly unfair it is – because it is. It just is.

*Alice Jolly is a novelist and playwright. In 2014 one of her short stories won the Royal Society of Literature's V.S. Pritchett Memorial Prize. She has written three books for Unbound. Her memoir,* Dead Babies and Seaside Towns, *won the PEN Ackerley Prize 2016. Her latest novel,* Mary Ann Sate, Imbecile, *was shortlisted for the Rathbones Folio Prize 2019, and her short-story collection,* From Far Around They Saw Us Burn, *was published in March 2023. She teaches creative writing at Oxford University.*

# Pronatalism and Me: Waking up from the Trance of Motherhood

*Jody Day*

When I was a girl, I wasn't particularly interested in dolls. If I did play with them, it was usually classroom enactments with me as their teacher or ones where we were all in a gang together, like Enid Blyton's Famous Five. Playing at being a mother wasn't part of my games, although perhaps that wasn't surprising, given that my own mother didn't make motherhood look like fun. A poorly mothered child herself, she'd had me as an unplanned teenage pregnancy and had later been married off to my violently abusive stepfather to give me 'a respectable home'. For us, family life was something to be endured, not enjoyed.

This was the 1970s, and second-wave feminism was really starting to have an impact on British society, generating opportunities for women that had been denied to my mother. She fervently encouraged me to embrace them. 'See the world and then settle down' and 'Never rely on a man!' were two statements that she drummed into me. Perhaps it's not surprising that the only doll I do remember being fond of was Air Hostess Barbie.

Reeling from the trauma of my childhood and with zero psychological language or awareness, I was determined not to have children. When I accidentally got pregnant at twenty, my world caved in. I was terrified of repeating my mother's and grandmother's story of having a baby young and 'ruining your life', and of mothering as I had been mothered. I chose to have an abortion and, although that turned out to be my only ever pregnancy, I don't regret it. My instinct had been right even if my information was patchy; I probably wouldn't have been able to be a 'good enough' mother without thera-peutic support – and at that time, I had no access to that. I didn't appreciate then that I wasn't condemned to repeat my mother's way of mothering because I was already conscious of it. I guess my mother didn't know that either; she was there with me when I had my termination and never once tried to persuade me against it.

At twenty-two I met my first husband and married him at twenty-six. I was still sure that I didn't want children and he was OK with that. At the time, I didn't know anyone else who thought the same, and I'd certainly never heard of the term 'childfree' or been exposed to anything other than the pronatalist – pro-birth – assumption that children were a 'when', not an 'if', and so I never really examined my think-ing around it. But after being a part of his large and loving family for several years, my idea of what 'family life' might mean began to shift. At twenty-nine, when our marriage was under stress due to the emergence of my husband's mental health difficulties, I changed my mind about having children. Everyone around us was having them and, after a lifetime of being considered different, for many reasons, including my upbringing, I longed to fit in. I thought that being a father would ground him and, while I hadn't yet done any healing work around my childhood, I felt like I could handle motherhood now.

My body had other ideas. After four years of trying for a baby, we started fertility investigations, but no reason for my inability to conceive was ever found. An operation to look around my uterus revealed no damage from the abortion, and we were just told to have 'lots of sex'. I was thirty-three, but no mention was made of the age of my eggs, or that we might want to consider fertility treatments. We continued to bumble along, my husband's mental health problems spilling over into alcoholism and addiction while I lost myself in baby-mania and co-dependency, rushing around London trying every possible quack cure to help us have a baby.

In my late thirties, my husband said that perhaps we should consider IVF and I realised with awful clarity that there was no way I wanted to bring a baby into the mess our life and marriage had become. Six weeks after that conversation, I had a nervous-breakdown-slash-spiritual awakening – thanks Brené Brown for that phrase – and our marriage fell apart. A scant year later we were divorced. It took my ex-husband ten awful years to get clean and, now in his sixties, he too mourns his childlessness, a grief that for many, many years I felt I carried alone.

With baby-mania in the driving seat, I pressed on, still unable to analyse what was really underneath my desperation to become a mother. I had a couple of post-divorce relationships in which we tried to get pregnant naturally, but I arrived at my mid-forties divorced, single, childless, broke and utterly lost. My friends had all either disappeared into motherhood or were still hoping to become parents. My career had sunk.

I'd lost my marriage, my peer group, my home, my savings, my mojo. I used to joke that the only invitations I ever got were to dental check-ups, but it was a hollow laugh at my own expense. I felt like social plankton, the bottom of the food chain, as though my only purpose in life was as a cautionary tale to younger women on how *not* to screw up their lives. After all I'd experienced, survived and achieved in my life, it seemed that nothing mattered either outwardly to society, or inwardly to my sense of worthiness, other than being a mother. I felt like a failed project, a failed woman, a failed human, and the world felt harsh and inhospitable in its judgement of me for getting this one basic thing so very, very wrong.

After a couple of years of intense loneliness and mental anguish, I started training to become a psychotherapist. While studying bereavement I realised that my despair had a name: grief. I was grieving my childlessness! Even though other people 'helpfully' told me that there was no way I could be grieving something I'd never had (and that *not* being a mother was amazing, so why wasn't I thrilled about it?), I immersed myself in grief studies. I began to realise that childlessness is a form of 'disenfranchised grief' – a term coined by the bereavement expert Dr Kenneth Doka in 1989 to describe a grief that it is not socially acceptable to experience or talk about. But even this could not explain why it was deemed OK to poke fun at my single self as being a 'crazy cat lady', or to simply ignore my existence altogether.

I was exhausted by trying to have conversations about my situation with people, therapists included, only to be met with comments such as 'children aren't all they're cracked up to be' or 'I guess you didn't really want them, or you would have adopted'. In 2011 I started a blog called Gateway Women, and soon strangers from all over the world were leaving comments that brought tears to my eyes – I wasn't alone after all. Here was proof that there really were other women having the same thoughts and experiences as me. I went from knowing no one who was childless-not-by-choice to finding and founding a community of women who 'got it'.

At that time, apart from a very small handful of married women blogging about life after failed infertility treatments (and who were very kind to me – thank you Pamela Mahoney Tsigdinos, Loribeth, and Lisa Manterfield), it was just me writing about being childless-by-circumstance or being both single and childless. I'm sad to say I was terrified that people would think I was 'one of those women who hate kids', which is what I'd internalised at the time about childfree-by-choice women, but ironically it was from childfree writers that I first learned why I felt this way. In 2012, Laura Carroll published her book on pronatalism, *The Baby Matrix*, and it rocked my childless world. It wasn't an easy read. At times I had the feeling I remembered from watching *Doctor Who* as a child, that I almost needed to hide behind the sofa and just peek over the top as I read it. In clear and irrefutable ways, it showed me that what I'd thought were 'my' ideas about womanhood and motherhood came from 'pronatalism': a very ancient idea but defined in 1974 by the childfree writers and advocates Ellen Peck and Judith Senderowitz as 'an attitude or policy that is pro-birth, that encourages reproduction, and exalts the role of parenthood'.

But what's wrong with being 'pro-birth', I hear you say? Surely that is a perfectly reasonable thing to be 'pro', isn't it? I mean, it's unlikely that very many readers of this book will be anti-natalist. Unfortunately, it's not quite that straightforward. The real sting in the tail is that pronatalism operates as a valuation system, one that glorifies parenthood (and motherhood especially) by *devaluing* non-parents, particularly non-mothers. It also affects mothers themselves by glossing over, or simply ignoring, the often heartbreaking challenges of maternity and motherhood. Pronatalism's call to bring babies into the world by any means possible is at odds with the level of support available for parents and children – let alone the adults they will become, and there are growing numbers of mothers who are prepared to admit (albeit mostly anonymously) that whilst they love their children, they deeply regret motherhood.

As well as setting up divides between women with and without children, pronatalism works to encourage children themselves to believe that having kids is the only socially acceptable way to be a proper grown-up woman. Notice how evil female characters in Disney films and fairy tales are never mothers or how, in adverts, apparently only mothers have worthwhile opinions. It's even in the language our government uses: how many times have you heard the phrase 'hard-working families' rather than 'households'? Pronatalism also promotes motherhood as easy, natural and instantly fulfilling, something which many mothers discover is far from the truth and yet which pronatalism encourages them to keep quiet about, lest they appear to be bad mothers.

Whilst learning all this woke me up from my baby-mania, it also revealed new layers of grief and shame because it forced me to reassess how much of my childless pain was truly *biological*, and to recognise that there was a huge social component too. I had to face up to the fact that because I hadn't understood how powerfully pronatalism had influenced my self-construct, I'd been denied a key piece of information that could have informed my actions through my fifteen years of trying to become a mother, and the heartbreak of letting that dream go.

There are so many 'mights' and 'could have dones' had I understood earlier the impact of living in a pronatalist society. I might have been much more curious about my ambivalence towards motherhood in my teens and twenties had I known the concept of being childfree existed, and might have felt drawn to that path as a valid and thought-through choice. I might have felt confident about examining the baby-mania that engulfed me in my thirties when my entire social group became one big kindergarten. And, as my then-husband and I went through a decade of trying to conceive, I might have been able to untangle the trauma of my unexplained infertility from the social stigma of possibly being childless, and made better sense of what was happening to me – to us. That awareness might even have saved our marriage because, despite our problems, in many ways we were very well suited and, with time and support, could have become a happy childless couple.

With an understanding of pronatalism, I might have been able to draw a line under my pursuit of motherhood after our divorce and could have begun my post-divorce life by focusing on personal healing and growth, rather than making it my goal to 'meet someone and do IVF'. But most of all, I might have been able to have a gentler, more conscious experience of coming to terms with motherhood being off the table. I might not have lost much of my forties – such a potentially powerful and productive decade – to grief and isolation. It would also have given me a better understanding of why people had such a problem with me not being a mother, and what might also have driven what I later termed the 'friendship apocalypse' of childlessness, and why people took issue with me talking and writing about my childlessness publicly. No one who knew me thought that using my real name and photo on my blog, or being interviewed in the media about my story, was a good idea. Not a single one.

Unbeknownst to me, pronatalism had been running, or ruining, my life for decades before I even knew the word. I felt humiliated that I had been so brainwashed and didn't even realise it. Where was my free will? What else had I been duped about? I really understood why Laura Carroll had used the analogy of the 'red pill' from *The Matrix* as part of her book – discovering the pronatalist 'matrix' that underpins our society shattered my assumptions about myself and the world. A line from the legendary feminist Gloria Steinem comes to mind: 'The truth will set you free, but first, it will piss you off!'

In the past decade, the conversation around childlessness has really grown in the UK and across the English-speaking world, and many have been kind enough to say that my work kindled that, even naming me as the 'founder of the childless movement' and, less often but more memorably, as 'the Beyoncé of childlessness'! Where once there was nothing, now there are so many podcasts, books, blogs, social media accounts and other brilliant things, including this collection of essays, that I can no longer keep up with them all.

However, I still feel that pronatalism, as both a word and a concept, is missing from many of our conversations (even spellcheckers don't recognise it!), and that until we include it, we will not begin to see the social change we long for in our families, friendships, partnerships, communities, organisations and societies. We are in the middle of a profound time in human history and, when the impact of population decline in the developed world starts to fully manifest, there may well be a hardening of attitudes against people without children and those ageing without children, whether we chose that life, or it chose us. I believe we've begun to see this recently in the US, with the rolling back of reproductive rights, and the UK, where significant newspapers such as the *Sunday Times* feel able to publish opinion pieces titled 'Should we tax the childless' that suggest the introduction of 'a negative child benefit tax for those who do not have offspring'.

Such kneejerk responses to demographic changes easily cast those without children as the problem, when in fact there are many ways that we can and do contribute to the culture and to civic society because we have the time, energy and education to do so. And we are happy to pay our taxes to support the services other people's children need, but we need to be valued for more than our economic function – we were each born childless and worthy, and we retain that intrinsic human worthiness whether we later have children or not.

The coming age needs everyone to be involved as our civilisation transforms through a time of radical change. I may not have biological children and grandchildren to worry about; my care and concern is broader: it is for *all* future generations. Pronatalism may say that because I'm neither a mother nor a grandmother my opinions and actions don't matter, that I don't have 'a real stake in the future', as the

Tory leadership candidate Andrea Leadsom once said of her opponent, Theresa May – we now hear the same from Elon Musk. But I disagree. I may be childless, but I can still be a good ancestor.

*Jody Day is the author of* Living the Life Unexpected: How to Find Hope, Meaning and a Fulfilling Future Without Children *and the founder of Gateway Women, the global friendship, support and advocacy network that has helped millions of women around the world to come to terms with involuntary childlessness. A psychotherapist and thought leader, she's also a volunteer ambassador for World Childless Week. She lives in rural Ireland, where she is working on a novel and nurturing her emerging 'Gateway Elderwomen' project. www.gateway-women.com*

# A 'Nearly Life'

*Rosie Wilby*

A familiar sad ache clawed at my insides. A recurring red stain in my pants. I was not pregnant. Again. But, unlike many of my straight friends, I was not tangibly trying to be. I just wished it so . . . somehow.

My girlfriend, Sarah, and I were nearly five years into a secret partnership. I was waiting for permission to lead my adult life, the one where we moved in together and had a family. A life that was culturally acknowledged by the traditional markers of weddings, honeymoons and holidays. Surely it was just around the corner. Her parents would eventually accept us as a couple, wouldn't they? After all, they had quite enjoyed the film *Brokeback Mountain* . . .

It was 2010. Civil partnerships had been available to same-sex couples in the UK for several years. And same-sex couples could now be recognised as legal parents of children conceived through the use of donated sperm, eggs or embryos. Yet these signs of progress felt a little too late for us. The damage had been done. Now perhaps only one painful thing still bonded Sarah and me: our common, unspoken yearning for the impossible – motherhood. How can you talk about

having a child together if you can't even talk about the relationship to anyone? Secrecy had catalysed our love's
exponential decay. We were so far beyond the starting line of
commitment yet had never even reached it.

Although we may have felt it, we were not alone. Many
had started out like us, with the same programming, the
relentless harmful messaging that turned any sort of real
future into a science fiction. Survival was a day-to-day concern and not a long-term project.

Coming out as a teenager back in 1988 had been so very
tightly wrapped up in a set of unbreakable assumptions: you
were an outsider, you could never marry, and most certainly
never become a parent.

My mum, unusually progressive for the times, told me all
about her own close female friendships. Perhaps she could
have been gay in a different era. She went to the library to
borrow books of lesbian poetry then recited from them at the
tea table. Yet amidst this excited frivolity came a sadder conclusion: 'I won't get any grandchildren, then.'

Margaret Thatcher's Conservative government had just
introduced Section 28 of the Local Government Act, which
outlawed the 'promotion' of homosexuality. IVF was only a
decade old.

When I graduated in the early 1990s and moved to London
to work in TV production, I started partying at gay clubs
and discovered an alternative sense of family that centred on
friendships rather than traditional models of marriage and
kids. Spending a thrilling decade embedded in a supportive
queer community where parenthood felt equally impossible
for all, I made peace with the prospect of never ever becoming a mum. We were mavericks and rebels. We broke free of

societal rules. And celebrated that freedom. As I once joked, 'Who cares about being left on the shelf when the shelf is piled high with drugs?'

I fell in love. I fell out of love.

Everything was fine.

I lost my mum.

Everything was not so fine.

Time to grow up.

And that's when I met Sarah. Whooosh. How many times had I said 'I love you' before this, before her? How could I say it differently now, add deeper resonance, reflect this new dimension, this extra universe of feeling that had snuck up and bolted itself onto my old version of love like a docking spaceship?

Surely this was my 'one', my soulmate: perhaps it was time to start imagining a future. Attitudes towards gay people had seismically shifted; I started to dream about our children and think, *what would they look like?* I even spoke onstage about hoodwinking my male comedy colleagues into donating sperm. Yet my hopeful dreams were punctured by waking to a nagging sadness that the world hadn't quite changed enough. Not for us. Not yet. The pressure was ultimately too much for Sarah. As the opening days of 2011 unfurled, and as the crackling and fizzing sounds of New Year fireworks had barely faded, I received a heartbreaking email. Our relationship had become just as impossible as our dreams of starting a family. We were over. If only things could have been different.

How can this form of grief, for someone or something that never existed, even be articulated? Do we even have a right to feel it when there is so much 'real' loss in the world? Perhaps it is time to give ourselves permission.

The Welsh language has a word that seems apt. *Hiraeth*

is a yearning which can be equated to homesickness. But a Welsh friend tells me, 'It's not necessarily for a home you actually had. It's a sense of not being in your right place, whatever that means to you.' Meanwhile the writer and artistic explorer Chris Ifso devised the concept of 'nearlyology' and wondered how the things that we nearly do can influence our lives and feelings. Perhaps my children are part of my 'nearly life'. The unfulfilled possibility of parenthood.

It was only really in 2017, when I began hosting a weekly radio show alongside my friend, the actor and musician Heather Peace, that I felt that gay parenthood was suddenly a reality in my immediate personal world. Heather was pregnant with twins, having already had one daughter with her wife Ellie. Just like me, she describes coming out as a teenager as having been 'tinged with sadness' due to the assumption that it meant 'giving up on having family and kids'. At forty-two, she was considered a geriatric mum. I was four years older, and I'd only just met my new partner, Suzanne. The timing didn't seem quite right to suddenly start talking babies. I was happy for Heather, and happy that the world was changing. But it was bittersweet. I felt like I had only just missed out on my chance of parenthood. As it happens, Suzanne became my wife and we have discovered a sense of family with our dog and cat. They're our children now.

One particular friend of mine was more fiercely determined than I to find a route to motherhood against all odds. When Fran was in her late thirties and struggling to meet a woman to settle down with, she decided to embark on the IVF journey on her own. She had a number of failed attempts and a miscarriage and describes the process as an emotional rollercoaster. When she hit forty, her fertility levels decreased. She pinned all her hopes on one last embryo, her final shot. It was a success, and she loves being a mum. However, she thinks that it is difficult to find a place where you can feel like you really belong when you're constantly 'surrounded by heteronormative families'. Other friends have fallen into parenting later in life by becoming involved with women who had previously had children during heterosexual marriages. They describe these new connections with their stepchildren as 'amazing'.

However LGBTQ people go about becoming parents, it is still uncommon. Yet as Heather points out, 'It can't happen by accident, so every child that comes into one of our relationship setups is madly, madly wanted.' For years I still wondered about Sarah, our split too acrimonious to remain friends. Yet one day, to my great shock, I heard that she had died. She had eventually been accepted by her family and had been surrounded by loved ones. Our 'nearly life' felt even more distant. It was not meant to be. The mental images of our children faded.

If I could travel back through time and give advice to my younger self, I would probably say, 'Parenthood will be possible for gay people. But only just in time for you. You'll have to be a bit of a pioneer and make some brave choices. But things are changing. You have more agency than you think you have.' Perhaps these words could have altered how I calibrated my choices around motherhood. I'll never really know. And, though it is hard sometimes, I can live with the not-knowing.

*Rosie Wilby is an award-winning comedian, author, speaker and the creator of global hit podcast and book* The Breakup Monologues.

# The Unspoken Trauma of Almost-Motherhood

## *Noni Martins*

At every family gathering since we got married in 2018, the women have asked me, 'How is married life?' followed by, 'Where are the babies?' We have been trying for a baby for almost six years; naturally for the first two and a half, and then, after a diagnosis of male factor infertility from my husband's years on dialysis following kidney failure when he was twenty-two, through IVF.

Once, at my mother's house, her friend assumed that, because I was wearing a kaftan, I must be pregnant. I didn't feel upset – in fact, I couldn't stop laughing as my mother turned my kaftan into a fitted dress to emphasise my 'no belly'. Later, I realised that I was laughing to mask the shock. Being African – my family is Zimbabwean, my husband's is Nigerian – there is a culture of respect, especially towards your elders. I didn't know how else to respond.

The women in our lives mean well; they want to be encouraging about having babies, and this is how they communicate it. It never feels like the right time for me to educate people on infertility when there's a whole culture to dismantle, and besides, I don't always have the emotional capacity to educate. Laughing it off is sometimes an act of self-care. A discussion like that can give you more hurt than you bargained for.

In fact, I find it very difficult to be 'not pregnant'. There is something impossible in trying to reconcile being an IVF patient with the fact that others are having babies naturally, just. LIKE. *THAT!* Your friends, people you know, strangers: it's everywhere. Don't get me wrong, I am very happy for my friends when they fall pregnant, carry to full term, and give birth to healthy babies, but each natural pregnancy I see or hear about is a reminder that I am not a mum yet and that I won't be able to fall pregnant naturally. It is heartbreaking. That is not an intention to take away from someone else's joy, rather a strong realisation of the lack of it in my own life.

When you are trying for a baby, the thing so many of us do is *keep it moving*. I had kept going, from trying to conceive naturally to having fertility treatment, without ever stopping to really take stock of what I had been through. The thing about IVF is that it's very scientific, and when something is that precise, we perceive the outcome as guaranteed. Imagine trying to get something for years and repeatedly getting nothing – there is no emotional training for this.

In fertility treatment, striking the balance between being hopeful and realistic is like trying to match the colours on a Rubik's Cube – possible, but also impossible. Once an embryo is implanted into your womb, you are classed as 'pregnant until proven otherwise', or PUPO. That kind of language is hard to detach from, even after a negative pregnancy test. You are left bewildered by it all. My second cycle was the first time that I really did feel PUPO, and for those ten days before testing I spoke to my belly with our baby's chosen name, and then had to grieve the loss of the possibility of loving that little person.

It has been incredibly difficult for me to process that I am nearing six years in this pursuit of motherhood and there is still no baby. I could process it initially after the first few months of trying, after a year, after two years, even, but when I started to realise that there is no guarantee of success, no matter how much I try, it really started to affect my mental health. I am traumatised by pregnancy tests now to the point that my husband has to buy them. I do not associate them with good news, or the heart-warming vibes I see in pregnancy-announcement videos. I don't have that experience; not even a 'maybe' or a faint line – always *not pregnant*.

In 2020, it hit me how much time I had lost to the tunnel-visioned 'trying to have a baby' thing. I did not know who I really was anymore. Without distractions during lockdown, I had become fully zoned in on baby-making to the point that, when a friend asked me, 'What have you done recently that has given you joy?' I couldn't answer. I simply could not remember the last time I had experienced something that made me feel joy. It was as though I had been on autopilot for years, heading towards one destination: motherhood. I was completely disconnected from the idea that life – even now, without a baby – still has meaning, and that there is a life to be lived even in the waiting.

On the few occasions that I have tried to explain to people that I am the way I am now because of trying to conceive and failing, people have always reduced it to one of two things. They either give me supposed reassurance that there is a time or reason for everything, or ask me why I want a baby. I find this last one particularly strange. I am not sure what it is about my being on a journey of this kind that makes people feel that I need to justify why I want to be a parent.

I don't think I necessarily want a baby more than a woman who falls pregnant quickly and naturally. When the journey is shorter, and not plagued by denial, displacement, disappointment and fertility treatments, you don't get to see the desire on display. I get the logic, but I cannot articulate enough the unsettling feelings of living in the in-between states of almost-motherhood. Not being a mother physically, but in constant pursuit of becoming one. No baby to show for that desire.

The trauma that is in my body now is not just about a baby; it's about everything. I have had PTSD-like responses to even the smallest things; to things that have been familiar to me my whole life – even to moments of joy. I am not entirely sure when it began, but I became plagued with an uneasiness that wouldn't go away. Was it one moment that changed everything, or was it a gradual build-up of the constant feeling of anxiety?

When our third round of IVF failed, the whole thing hit me like a bus. The crying caught me unawares; while I was drinking tea, while I was eating, while I was staring outside or staring at my phone, while I was driving. Tears rolled down my cheeks with no sound or body response at all, just a slow release of sadness. I told my husband that failed IVF felt like being in prison. Because of my good behaviour there was a plan to release me soon, but then the day came and I found out something unknown had sabotaged my case and I had to continue serving a life sentence.

I started having panic attacks – and I mean full-blown meltdowns. One incident that stands out is from a friend's thirtieth birthday, one of the best days we've had as a friendship group. We threw a surprise dinner party for her, and I drank, I danced, I laughed. I felt joyful. I was meant to spend four nights in London. Instead, when I woke up the next morning, I changed my train ticket and told everyone I was leaving. I couldn't explain why, not even to myself. I just needed to get home.

When I sat on the train at London Euston, I fell apart. I started crying, softly at first, then hysterically, and before I knew it I was heaving, dizzy and confused. I felt so vulnerable. It was as if the joy I had felt just the night before had to be met in equal measure by sadness. I felt it like a punch in my gut. In that moment, there was nothing I could do to make myself feel better.

Initially, I linked these attacks only with trying to conceive but I soon learned that one state of being eventually infiltrates all parts of one's life. You end up with a body that is a walking time bomb; what Bessel van der Kolk means in his book on trauma, *The Body Keeps the Score*. He describes how traumatised people feel unsafe, their bodies feeling under attack, as though the traumatic event is ongoing.

Myleene Klass said something in her 2021 documentary about miscarriage that really resonated with me: 'I've got my baby now, but God: I lost a lot of me.' There is an assumption that, once I have a baby, everything will return to 'normal'; that I will return to a former self; that just because I want a baby 'so much', it makes me immune to the psychological and physiological impact of being on this infertility journey. I don't doubt for a second that my pursuit of motherhood was the catalyst for my trauma, but it is not just about a baby anymore. One year, we took a break from trying, and it was as though the trauma had to manifest itself in other ways and through other aspects of my life.

It took a meltdown at Manchester Airport before I realised that trauma had consumed me. I remember my mother saying to me, 'I don't recognise you like this; this is not you, Noni.' I understood what my mother was saying because I also didn't recognise myself. I have not come out unscathed from this process. My brain has re-engineered itself to process the trauma, and my response mechanisms do not work in the same way they did five years ago.

I think the trauma is made worse because people don't really understand the gravity of the infertility experience. We censor women and men about the very real states of chaos that they might be feeling. When people ask me how I am, I always feel the pressure to make it seem less bad than it is because I know that they could not handle the truth if I were to speak it.

This journey has ruined my spirit and I am definitely not the person I used to be. There is no other way to articulate that. I am so exhausted from trying to censor my experience for everyone else's comfort. And I admit, much of it has been my own doing because I have always been the kind of person who struggles to be vulnerable. Even now, I rarely want to show how I feel; mainly because I hate the pity (or what I perceive as such) that can come from telling people you don't have children, and that you are struggling to have them. I usually get vacuous words of affirmation and the whole 'It's going to be OK!' narrative in response – but to be honest, it's not going to be OK. Even once the baby is here, even if the baby never comes. My life is forever changed by this process.

I only fully realised this after going to my GP (for something unrelated to fertility, for a change). This was the same GP who had so compassionately given us our male factor infertility diagnosis, who had seen me after each failed IVF cycle, and signed me off work after the third. She knew that my husband had a kidney transplant last year. And she had also referred me for a minor surgery, which did not cure the chronic pain I had suffered for years.

When she asked me how I was, I immediately started crying. Through hysterical tears, I said over and over, 'I feel so overwhelmed. I feel so overwhelmed.'

She looked at me with the sweetness of a mother. 'Are you suicidal?'

'No!' I was shocked that she asked me this, and again when she repeated it.

'Are you feeling suicidal, Noni? You have been through such a lot in such a short space of time. I am very worried about your mental wellbeing.'

I suppose that, from where she was sitting, it did seem as though I no longer had the will to live. The thing about living with trauma in your body is that you are always in fight, flight or freeze mode. I started to fully recognise the trauma I had been carrying because, while I was not suicidal, I didn't have a feeling of being *alive*. I had, as Bessel van der Kolk puts it, learned to hide from myself. I was numbing my awareness of what was going on inside me, the good as well as the bad, and, my goodness, I had been doing a lot of numbing: with alcohol; fleeting moments with friends and family; with TV; with distractions; with social media; even with my own @unfertility platform.

I had wanted to do something meaningful with my pain,

which is why I started my podcast and Instagram community. Because we live in a culture of toxic positivity, most people do the telling-my-story-publicly thing *after* the miracle, after the baby. I had been band-aiding my trauma with false reassurances while dismissing the very real negative emotions that I felt. But repurposed pain is still pain, and sometimes the only meaningful thing you need to be working on is yourself.

As women, and especially Black women, we fall into these superwoman 'I can endure anything!' narratives so easily, but IVF has shown me just how important it is to be a bit selfish. Navigating treatment in tandem with normal life gets so overwhelming, and I am constantly feeling like I cannot catch a break. If it's not a work deadline, it's an appointment, an injection, or being a loving wife, daughter, sister. It's looking after the home, the puppy; it's feeling so sick on the medications, the side effects; it's friends and family still expecting 100 per cent from you.

One gift that has come from this process is that the trauma forces me to feel. I've learned that, when the panic attacks come, there is nothing I can do to stop them. They only stop when I resist fighting, and just feel it out. Even past traumas that I had learned to live with: my trauma forces me to feel those too and now it's like I'm starting all over again. It has forced me to feel, even in the most awkward situations. Most of my panic attacks have been in public. I remember a lady sitting next to me and asking me with real concern if I wanted to talk about it. It's funny to me now, but at the time I felt so distressed that she had felt compelled to offer compassion and a listening ear.

I have learned to give myself permission to cry. I have a

rule now that I allow my body to release in this way so that it does not 'keep the score' and send me into a cumulative meltdown. My husband has had to get used to very random thirty-second cries that seem to come from nowhere, and having to reconcile that with the fact that I might then be laughing or debating passionately about something interesting the next minute.

Everyone handles grief differently. What I know now is that I am in no position to be responsible for the feelings of others. The person I really need to focus on is myself. I don't know what the future holds for me, but for now, I'm still a mama-in-waiting. And I'm hoping and healing at the same time.

*Noni Martins is the founder of* Unfertility, *a three-pronged podcast, community and awareness campaign that seeks to break the silence, stigma and shame around unconventional fertility journeys through the voices of Black women, including her own.*

# Small, Soft, Grey Pig

*Laura Barton*

I

Some things I keep:

A collection of pregnancy tests, lines long faded.
A small, soft, grey pig, who sat in the window of a children's
store in New York.
A bib I bought in California, the year before beginning IVF.

Also:

A selection of crystals, in various shades of pink, blue, white
and green. One for every baby lost.

They lie in the dark of my bedside cabinet. Peculiar relics of
a different time.

Some days I take them out, and sit with them: the small, soft,
grey pig in my hands, the bib that still smells faintly of America, the crystals bought one sad, hot afternoon in Los Feliz,

in an act of desperation. Not that I place any faith in crystals. Not that I recall, now, their specific powers or promises. But because I needed to turn each loss into something beautiful I could hold.

II

To lose a baby is a reckoning with absence; with the space that opens up before you, vast and quiet and empty.

People give you things to make it better. One partner gave me lingerie. Another brought a pomegranate and a copy of *National Geographic*. Friends sent flowers and cards and chocolates, and, once, a ceramic tile that read: 'Your button fell off but I picked it up and sewed it back on again.'

I thought about that a lot. The button that fell, that could not be sewn back. I thought about it so much that I put the tile away in a box where I could not see it. Meanwhile the *National Geographic* went unread. The knickers unworn. I let the pomegranate rot.

I am confused, even now, by my adamant rejection of these gifts. Perhaps I deemed their consolation too clumsy, an affront to the delicacy of this particular kind of grief. Perhaps I was angry with the world. Perhaps I did not want to be touched.

There is already a great intangibility to pregnancy. The body swells, the belly, the breasts, but the baby itself remains curiously abstract. There on the sonographer's scan, a strange constellation, a creature of the deep. In the outside world, we measure its gathering size through approximation to familiar objects: a poppy seed, a blueberry, an apricot, a grapefruit. When a pregnancy fails, it is hard for anyone not carrying that hypothetical grapefruit, that half-pictured poppy seed, to feel its loss with any keenness, to understand the sudden monstrous absence.

The days that followed my last miscarriage were filled with mute and dutiful industry; the steady erasure of something already invisible. The text to cancel the morning's midwife visit. The ultrasound appointment crossed from the calendar. Wiping clean the Google searches for baby slings and clothes for newborns. On a grey spring morning, folding away the one maternity dress I had bought, and had yet to wear, but that had hung on the door of my wardrobe, like a promise.

And when it was done, I sat alone in the bath and cried.

The year rolled on, my due date passed, another childless autumn came and went. The days were pale and cold. I avoided friends, family, my godchildren. I could not find the words to express my loss. Everything was blank. Everything was space.

## III

When you have lost many babies, or struggled with fertility, it is easy to sentimentalise the objects you have accumulated along the way. Still I keep the assorted paraphernalia of two rounds of IVF: needles, syringes, small vials of medication; the printed-out instructions of my treatment plan and dosage; the photographs of sperm donors, whose faces I had studied so closely. They sit in a zip-up cooler bag, given to me by a clinic in Crete. On its side, in green felt-tip pen, my name and contact details written in Greek.

I suppose it is strange to find comfort in the things that represent such resounding failure, but to me these objects have been something like companions; the only true witnesses to this intimate struggle.

On the morning I learned that my last round of IVF had been unsuccessful, I walked through my house still carrying my negative pregnancy test, to sit at my desk and be interviewed for a radio programme about the economics of the music industry.

Later, when the show aired, I heard my voice carried through the speakers, talking warmly of streaming figures and the emotional value of songs. I laughed at points. I sounded engaged. But I remembered how, as I talked, I had held onto the slim plastic test, tight in my palm, as if to stop my heart from buckling.

## IV

I used to say I wanted six children. I was a child myself, then, and this was a storybook number. Everything I dreamed of was boundless: a large house, a garden that ran down to a lake, a joyous, sprawling family.

Later, I settled on four.

Later still, I hoped for one.

And in the gap now forged between the imagined life and the real, I have a sense of having misplaced the life I thought I would live.

It is hard to break the habits of thought, to stop my mind from wandering to versions of the future that will now never be: the world I wanted to show my children, the stories I wanted to tell them, the intricate decisions I had made regarding diet, schooling, travel. There is a corner of my brain that still pictures myself long-married, settled, content, quite besotted with my grandchildren, even if the arithmetic shows me the impossibility of this scene.

Some long nights I lie awake and wonder what will happen to the things I own: all my books, all my pictures, all my records; the dresses that my mother gave to me, that I hoped I might pass to my own daughter; my great-aunt's powder bowl and hat collection, the tablecloth she crocheted just for me, the nursing chair with the embroidered back. And it is strange to conclude that after me, there will be no one left to feel tender towards these objects.

V

When you reach the other side of it all, after the years of losing babies and the rounds of fertility treatment, you come to see how your relationship with yourself and your body has grown distorted and odd. You have been examined, inspected and scanned, your ovaries measured, your fallopian tubes checked, your blood tested over and over. You worry about the things you eat and drink and do. You worry about the things you don't. You take supplements, inject yourself with hormones, pay for acupuncture and therapy. And at the end of it all, you feel less of a person and more like a vessel. An object. A thing.

But you are a thing, now, that does not quite fit. That is a problem.

People give you things, once again, to make it better. They invite you to spend time with their children, they make you a godmother, you become the strange extra limb at family dinners. Sometimes, after a glass of wine, they will even give you advice, offer their sperm, their husband's sperm. 'Maybe,' they will say, 'you just need to relax. Stop worrying!' There is always some story of a distant friend who finally conceived after simply giving up, and having fun.

At some point, they will let their voice turn low and sombre and ask: 'Have you thought about adoption?' This has become my least favourite of all the questions. Of course I have thought about adoption. I have thought about it often. I have investigated the process, which is long and complicated, especially if you are single. And oh God, I am tired.

I hate this question mostly because of its desire for neatness, because somewhere within it lies the belief that the world must add up, that the parentless be united with the childless, no loose ends left. It is the fertility equivalent of matchmaking.

Sometimes, after a couple more glasses of wine, they will drop their voices further and confess that they aren't entirely sure they like being parents. 'Don't do it,' they say. 'Maybe you're better off! Look at the life you have! The freedom!'

It doesn't always feel like freedom. Most days it feels like absence. It feels like nothing you can hold on to. No dry land.

## VI

Some days I think about a card that came with flowers sent by an ex-boyfriend, absent when I miscarried, and that the florist miswrote, so its message appeared garbled and strange. I think about what he meant to say, and the words that were missing. I think about how he was missing. I think about how the baby was lost.

In recent times I have learned to sit in absence. Not to fill or fix what isn't there, just to let the grief roll in, to feel the waves of it.

I am there on the edge of my bed, with the small, soft, grey pig in my hands, and the bib that still smells faintly of America, and the crystals in pink, blue, white and green. We are holding each other, these objects and I. We are holding each other, until the loss turns into something beautiful.

*Laura Barton is a writer and broadcaster. A feature writer and music columnist for the* Guardian *for more than a decade, she now writes for a variety of publications. Her first novel,* Twenty-One Locks, *received a Betty Trask Award. She is a regular contributor to Radio 4 and Radio 3, and since 2018 she has curated the literary stage at the Green Man Festival. She also moonlights in A&R for a music publishing company and has signed some of contemporary music's most sought-after acts.*

# Society

# A Historical Perspective on Women Without Children

*Emma Duval*

When I envision a childless woman, I see a figure in the distance. While I picture her alone, I know she is not lonely. Even if she might seem weary, she stands tall. I imagine that she has a rich inner world from which she draws her strength, and no matter how wounded she feels, she holds space for others. Unfortunately, that is not how society sees her. A woman's purpose has historically been tied to her ability to bear children, so women without children have been portrayed as cursed, faulty and unworthy. They have been described in hurtful terms and judged in every and any part of their lives for their childlessness. As I have found through my work researching women without children for my Instagram account, @millennialemma, negative perceptions have spread through the centuries via literature, religion and medical science. This has resulted in an accumulation of stereotypes and prejudice that unfairly compares women based on whether they are mothers.

Through my research, I found that signs of this collective prejudice are especially visible in the lives of royal women, for whom not having children wasn't simply an intimate subject between husband and wife but a political matter with ramifications for the ruling dynasty. These women's bodies became the centre of public discourse and, if they couldn't fulfil their duty of providing an heir, they faced humiliation, rejection and public scrutiny.

Mary Tudor, the daughter of Henry VIII and sister to Elizabeth I, was taunted for her childlessness. She had exhibited visible signs of pregnancy which led her and others to believe that she was with child but went months past her due date without giving birth, a situation which became the subject of increasingly scandalous gossip. Her phantom pregnancies were a source of great physical and emotional distress; a trauma compounded by the public humiliation she suffered, including with pamphlets implying that anyone would be foolish to believe that she would ever give birth, unless it was – perhaps as punishment for her sins – to a monstrous creature.

While Mary Tudor was judged by the public, the main source of abuse for a childless wife was often her own husband. The medieval queen Teutberga was increasingly mistreated by her husband Lothair II, king of Lotharingia, who wanted to marry his mistress, Waldrada, who was the mother of his illegitimate son. Lothair first sought an annulment (which wasn't granted) before resorting to accusing Teutberga of incest with her brother Hucbert and forcefully imprisoning her. Her ordeal only ended with Lothair's unexpected death in 869, after which she spent her remaining years in an abbey, having hopefully found some peace.

Because royal marriages were first and foremost political tools, some might overlook the way that Mary Tudor and Teutberga were treated for their childlessness, seeing it as a mere consequence of the ruthless world of monarchs. However, even royal unions based on love could break under the weight of childlessness, and once-devoted husbands could suddenly become bitter and resentful, as Joséphine de Beauharnais ultimately found. When Napoléon Bonaparte first fell in love with her, she was already an older widow with two children from her previous marriage. The future French emperor was so passionately in love that he disregarded social conventions and married her. However, his strong affection was apparently not enough to sustain a childless marriage: Bonaparte rejected Beauharnais and eventually had the marriage annulled because of her perceived barrenness. He remarried with the primary intention of having children, showing little care for the individuality of his next wife, Marie-Louise of Austria, by stating, 'I am only marrying a womb.'

The portrayal of women without children as objects of pity and desolation is so common in literature that we might not even realise it. In *Metamorphoses*, the Roman poet Ovid detailed childlessness as weaponised by a mother who, boasting of having more children than her rival, describes the other mother as having barely avoided the 'childless woman's shame'. Phrased to purposefully inflict pain and humiliation on the other woman by questioning her fertility, those few words reveal a lot about the hierarchy of women within society: from the woman without any children at the bottom, to the woman with the most children at the top.

The inferior status of non-mothers compared to mothers is found in literary works across the globe. In his poem 'The Deserted Wife' (here translated by Anne Birrell), the third-century Chinese poet Ts'ao Chih described a childless woman as a star who loses its shine and dies in the darkness:

*With child she is the moon that sails the skies,*
*Childless she's like a falling star.*
*Skies and moon each wax and wane,*
*A falling star dies without a glimmer.*

The beautiful imagery does little to soften the caustic perception of childlessness, especially in its comparison to the glow of motherhood. Once again, it's not just that women are judged based on their maternal status, but that the woman without children finds herself to be the most aggrieved party.

Centuries later, the French author Victor Hugo, when writing about a young Cosette in his novel *Les Misérables*, would very matter-of-factly state that 'a little girl without a doll is almost as unhappy, and quite as impossible, as a woman without children'. Why did Hugo choose that specific comparison when there are so many metaphors one could think of to describe the sadness of that little girl? Perhaps because motherhood is viewed as a woman's highest desire, reflected early in her childhood through her playing with dolls. Therefore, according to that viewpoint, without a doll or a baby, the female figure finds herself to be profoundly distressed.

Fairy tales and folklore have long cast older women without children in a negative light; as witches that might harm children or as desperate women who will steal them. Lady Jane Wilde documented one such saying in her 1888 book on Irish superstition: 'Beware of a childless woman who looks fixedly at your child.' Over the generations, such stories have entrenched the idea of the woman without children as a wicked or pitiful figure in our collective unconscious.

It's certainly been upheld by various religions, including Christianity, Judaism and Islam, as demonstrated by the pressure women from those religious communities still face today. The Book of Genesis in the Bible relates how Adam and Eve were ordained by God to 'be fruitful and multiply'. Consequently, fertility and infertility became weighted representations of faith, with the belief that personal sins or a lack of faith were the cause of any childlessness. In the Bible, women who experience infertility, barrenness or childlessness eventually become mothers if they remain faithful to God. This is the case for the matriarch of the Abrahamic religion, Sarah, the wife of Abraham, who is childless until she is blessed by God, at age ninety, with the birth of her son Isaac. Two generations later, when Rachel, the wife of Isaac's son Jacob, gives birth to a son after struggling with infertility, she states that 'God has taken away my disgrace', a clear expression of the inherent stigma of childlessness. Although these stories are used to help women without children through their grief, the correlation between faith and fertility, and the fact that childlessness as a permanent situation is never presented in these texts, can be especially damaging to those experiencing prolonged or lifelong childlessness.

Permanent childlessness is, however, found in Islam, specifically in the life of Aisha, one of the most notable wives of the Prophet Muhammad. A childless widow and a revered figure in Islam, her story should have inspired compassionate attitudes towards other women without children. Yet, demeaning beliefs, such as that 'a straw mat [thrown] in a corner of the house is better than a barren woman', can be found in some *hadith* (a transmission of religious guidance based on what the Prophet reportedly said, did, or approved of). This dichotomy between the glorification of the childless Aisha and the objectification of the anonymous barren woman might seem surprising, but it's simply representative of the unique position of Aisha within the Muslim faith as a woman above reproach and an outlier in many ways compared to ordinary women. The place of non-mothers remains, at best, an afterthought – an inconvenient reality for the congregation and religious leaders.

In the 1800s, physicians overwhelmingly blamed a couple's infertility on women. Writing in the *Obstetric Gazette* in 1883, H. R. Bigelow confidently referred to women's pursuit of higher education or their participation in the women's suffrage movement as 'self-caused conditions' of their sterility. While it might seem like satire to today's readers, those theories were accepted as factual and scientific; after all, physicians – and especially obstetricians – were supposed to have the highest level of expertise and knowledge about the human body. Although long since disproven, these beliefs have anchored themselves in the general population's consciousness, hints of which can still be sensed today, such as when women seeking fertility treatments are offered unsolicited advice from family and friends about what they might be doing 'wrong'. (It is now generally recognised that the cause of infertility is divided fairly evenly between men and women.)

If being involuntarily childless was seen as a pitiful situation, what of the childfree – those who purposefully chose not to have children? They certainly faced much contempt and disdain. Examples of the disproportionate anger expressed towards voluntarily childless women as 'selfish, vain, silly, heartless creatures, who do not merit the name of woman' can be found in late nineteenth-century literature (that charming line is from Fanny Aikin Kortright's 1869 anti-suffragist argument, *Pro aris et focis*).

Then, at the turn of the twentieth century, declining birth rates among white women fuelled the xenophobic and racist concept of 'race suicide' – similar to the 'great replacement' conspiracy theory promoted by the white nationalist far right today. This led to feverish calls to increase birth rates and the further vilification of voluntarily childless (white) women, including by US president Theodore Roosevelt, who publicly decried what he considered to be the 'viciousness, coldness, shallow-heartedness, self-indulgence' of (white) women who wilfully abstain from motherhood. Those same irrational fears and today's declining birth rates have ignited a similarly abject fire in the hearts of many politicians and public figures, whose solutions range from taxing the childless (financial pressure) to stripping away reproductive rights (forced motherhood and loss of bodily autonomy). For generations of women like me, who grew up after the women's liberation movement secured many of the rights we might take for granted, a dystopian future awaits us if we don't fight back. Worse, in some countries, such as the USA and Poland, these basic reproductive rights have already been regressing or dismantled in recent years.

While it might feel overwhelming to realise the extent to which not having children is considered an undesirable state of life, this overview is not meant to sound hopeless. On the contrary, it is meant to spark in each reader a burning desire to reject the status quo; it is meant to help women without children realise that any feelings of guilt, shame or self-blame are the result of centuries of indoctrination and should be denounced as such. It is also meant to harness the power of women's history, not just to show the many ways that childless women have been wronged, but also to find strength from those who have advocated in favour of a more positive perception of women without children.

Childless relatives have often been involved in the lives of their nieces and nephews; shaping their character, encouraging interests, and providing some additional attention and care. While they might not be the child's primary caregiver, they are able to create a unique bond – perhaps in part because their childlessness affords them to be more available to other people's children. In 1960, *The Atlantic* featured a column from the then-editor Edward Weeks on his unmarried and childless aunt, Eliza Gracie Suydam. 'Aunt Liz' was a key figure in his family and evidently much loved. Weeks' affectionate tribute ended with a question: 'How can you thank a person as selfless as that, a maiden aunt, for bringing out the self-confidence, the loyalty, the resourcefulness you never knew you possessed?' Like Weeks, I have been profoundly influenced by relatives and family friends who had no children. Society might not appreciate or recognise the important role these women played in my life, but I do.

One of the leaders of the women's suffrage movement in the nineteenth century, Elizabeth Cady Stanton, openly reproached the fact that only wives and mothers were being valued by society. Referencing her contemporaries, the social reformer Susan B. Anthony and the sculptor Harriet Hosmer, women who 'have done great things in the world without having borne children', she effectively advocated for the recognition and respect of single women without children. This is especially notable since Stanton herself was married with seven children – a situation which placed her in an elevated position within society but restricted her in-person involvement in the women's rights movement. Because of her responsibilities towards her husband and children, she had to remain at home, where she wrote speeches that were delivered by Susan B. Anthony, who, as a single woman without children, had the freedom to travel.

Identifying themselves as 'a childless woman' or 'a childless wife', some women also wrote open letters which appeared in the press. In response to Theodore Roosevelt's previously mentioned comments on the duties of (white) women to procreate, an American woman wrote anonymously to defend herself for not having children. In the heartfelt and powerful essay 'Why I Have No Family', published in the New York *Independent* in 1905, she detailed her reasons for choosing not to have any children, from the relatively common risk of dying during childbirth to the impact that motherhood would have on her work, her marriage, and her own financial independence. Addressing many concerns which still preoccupy women today, she vehemently denied 'the right of any one to criticise me who is not doing something to lighten the pressure' imposed on women, and especially mothers. Such feelings are still being vocalised today, as the demands of motherhood remain difficult to balance for most women, largely due to structural issues we all face in this flawed patriarchal and capitalist system. In a way, the issues faced by non-mothers and mothers are simply opposite sides of the same coin, which is why reciprocal support over shared struggles – and not divisiveness over perceived differences – is necessary.

Whether you identify as childless, childfree, or any

variation of 'mother' – including spiritual, substitute, or symbolic – I hope that you will feel a burning desire to reject society's perception of women without children as objects of pity or contempt. Only by advocating for ourselves and for others can we hope to improve how the vast spectrum of childlessness is presented, and therefore how women without children are perceived and treated. It's time for more dignified representation. It's time to change the narrative.

*Emma Duval is a writer and the founder of the Childfree History Museum, the first virtual museum dedicated to the history of women without children. Through her Instagram account @millennialemma, she amplifies positive representation of childfree, childless and single women.*

# The Silence of Shame

*Yvonne John*

I guess I'll start by telling you who I am now. Today, I am a
Badass Warrior Queen! I laugh at myself when I say this
because it's taken me so long – so much soul-searching,
letting go of shame, (self) forgiveness, self-care and self-
acceptance – to be able to see myself as this incredible person
who has achieved so much.

There are still times when I can't believe that I am here and
times when I question how I got here in the first place, but I
am, and I did. It's taken me so long to see myself this way
because for as long as I can remember I have been underesti-
mated, criticised and put down.

Not only was I told as a young woman that I needed to be
'better' than my white counterparts thought of me, I was also
told that I needed to follow a traditional, acceptable path in
terms of my education (going to university), my career (I was
to be a doctor, a lawyer or even a shop assistant, depending
on who I was speaking to at the time), my marriage (to a
Dominican) with the children to follow, and it had to be in
that order.

I did accomplish a few things off that list: I graduated

from university and became a biomedical scientist (BMS or medical laboratory scientific officer as it was known back then). I remember one of my old teachers questioning how I got onto the course, as it sounded 'too good' for me – they had thought I'd be a shop assistant, of course. I got my first proper job as a biomedical scientist in a London hospital straight out of university and got married many years later. I did this all in the correct order. OK, there were some blips along the way, but who has a smooth life journey? The important thing is that I did what was expected of me – so why didn't the children follow?

After graduating and getting my first job (I'll leave the difficulties I faced at that point in my life to another time), I was on my way to getting that career that I had heard so much about. It wasn't what my dad had prescribed, but I guess being a scientist was a good (enough) alternative. So, on to step two, looking for a husband (imagine me singing these words). To be honest, marriage was the furthest thing from my mind. Being in my early twenties and a newly qualified BMS, I wanted to travel and see the world, which I did, much to my parents' disapproval. They couldn't comprehend why I would leave a 'good job' to go travelling. I loved visiting new countries, experiencing different cultures and collecting the most amazing memories with every place I visited. Dating, on the other hand, was another story. That quest to find the husband I was expected to marry was going to be harder than I had imagined.

Looking back, I realised that no one ever talked to me about dating, what to look for in a prospective partner or husband, or even about knowing and loving myself. I found myself searching in the dark, going from one disappointingly painful relationship to another. On reflection, I realised that I didn't know (or even like) myself well enough to know what I deserved, and I certainly lacked the confidence to be OK with saying no. In my head, if I said no, 'they' (men) wouldn't like me, and if they got to know me, they would leave, so I was constantly changing in the hope that I would be liked and accepted. My terminations are a reminder of the shy, easily intimidated younger me who just wanted to be loved.

My second pregnancy and termination was the one that floored me. Neither pregnancy was planned. I wasn't in a relationship with either man, and I certainly wasn't with someone who cared about me, let alone cared about what I did. Neither of those men seemed bothered that I was pregnant, which influenced my decision not to keep the baby. I really couldn't bring myself to have this lifelong attachment to these men, let alone be a single mum, which, to me, seemed like the biggest taboo for a twenty-something black woman. I did secretly wish that man number two had asked me to keep the baby. I really liked him, but he wasn't available to be in a relationship with me.

At that time, I berated myself for making this mistake, not once but twice. For being stupid enough to be there. I remember how deep the feeling of shame was. I couldn't even look at my reflection in the mirror. I walked down the street with my head held low, hiding from the gazes that would know what I had done if they looked into my eyes. I remember telling myself that it would be OK because one day someone would love me enough to want to have a child with me. That day never came.

I didn't really grow up with the desire to be a mum; I grew up with the expectation that I would be one. Other than hearing that I'd have babies with Down's syndrome if I left it too late, or that my biological clock was ticking, I never really thought about my fertility at all. It was obviously on other people's minds though, as I heard all about the expectations they had for my womb. Having a family just wasn't on my radar. Children seemed to be other people's dream and not mine.

There were times in my twenties when I had thoughts of having a child, usually driven by the fact that whoever I was dating had nice hair or nice eyes, or looked good in a suit. I remember one guy wanting to have a child with me because 'we would have good-looking babies', but that didn't seem to be enough to get me off the ambivalence train. Away from these thoughts, and the pressures of belonging to a church with a 'no sex before marriage' rule, having children was the furthest thing from my mind, even though I assumed I could if I wanted to. No one told me that 'it' may not happen.

I was thirty-seven when I met my now ex-husband. It was an easy yes when he proposed, and I married at thirty-nine. While we were dating, we had talked about having kids and agreed that we weren't bothered; he because of his age, and me because I felt that I had made my choices. This ambivalence stayed with me until I hit forty, so it surprised us both when I brought up the idea of having a baby. I guess that I got caught up in the euphoria of being happily married (OK OK, give me a break, I didn't think I'd ever get married – well, no one did, so let me have this one). Looking back on this, I see how flippant I was being about the whole thing. Even then, I was still brushing off the possibility of it not happening with the idea that we'd still be OK because at least 'we tried'.

My unexplained infertility diagnosis sent me emotionally over the edge. I instantly knew that I wouldn't become a mum, but what I was unprepared for was the tsunami of grief that followed. All of a sudden, I couldn't be around my friends and their young children. This was so unexpected. It felt like yesterday I was OK, and today life felt unbearably shit! I'd be around them and their mum friends with the sudden urge to run out of the house and cry. I'd want to get off the train after watching young families meet up for a day out in London. Tears would sting my eyes as I watched a woman interacting with her son, the cutest of the cute, knowing that I would never have these moments with my children. Hearing my dad telling stories, with a glint in his eye, of his grandkids and what they got up to broke me from the inside out, as I realised that he would never have stories to tell about my kids.

I never got to experience the joy of being pregnant, of celebrating that 'we' had conceived a child, along with the hopes and dreams that come in that moment. Is it a boy or a girl? What will they look like? Who will they take after? What will they be when they grow up? I had secretly hoped for a girl, imagining her crawling onto her father's lap while he read and, later, us two ganging up on him, joining together in the solidarity of girl power. I never got to dream about my child. I never got to experience that look of pride from my then husband because I was carrying his child.

Unexplained infertility left me with the debilitating shame of my past terminations, along with the resentment, anger and hurt of trying to conceive in my marriage, the scars of which will always remain in my heart. I hated hearing people telling me that my infertility 'was God's will', or that 'I'll pray for you', 'God knows best' and 'have faith'. I took all that to mean that God didn't think I deserved to be a mum.

Finding Jody Day's Plan B programme and the Gateway Women community gave me the opportunity to understand what I was experiencing. This all-consuming sadness (it took me a while to accept this as grief) surprised me because of my past ambivalence. I was able to look my (in)fertility journey in the eye, along with the dark stuff that had essentially been buried for years. I questioned why I wanted children and why I had said no to motherhood in my twenties. I questioned the cultural narrative that was present in my life, and most poignantly, I wrote a letter to my younger self forgiving her. I told her that I knew she hadn't made a mistake and that I understood her choices were made from love to protect her unborn children. My younger self wanted better for them, more than I could have given them back then. This helped me to reconcile the fragmented parts of me and to start the healing process. Facing my grief helped me own my story and find my voice, a voice that had been silenced for so long. Shame is such a debilitating bitch!

My feelings about myself are very different today. I'm not sure if the negative voice ever goes entirely, but it is much quieter. Now I realise that I *am* amazing and I see this in so many ways. I was never taught about self-care, but how I present myself now is part of it for me – I feel every bit the Badass Warrior Queen with the clothes I wear. Taking long baths, watching what I eat and who I surround myself with, and trying to be better at setting boundaries are all elements of self-care for me. This reappraisal also helped me learn that what people think about me usually reflects who they are and where they are at in life.

The first time that I felt unapologetically me in public was speaking at an International Women's Day event in 2017. I thought that I was going to die as I hyperventilated, waiting for my turn to get on that stage. I thought that everyone would hate me when they knew my truth – and that they certainly would not accept my grief around not becoming a mother because I gave up that chance many years before. I even struggled with telling this part of my story when I was writing my book, but it felt disingenuous to leave it out when it was the reason why I struggled with my grief and why I felt that I didn't deserve to grieve in the first place. My abortions are a part of who I am, and if I was going to speak, I needed to be heard for all that I am. I took a deep breath, walked onto that stage, opened my mouth, and showed the world my scars.

Something inside me knew that I needed to speak up, but what kept driving me forward then was the responses: 'Me too.' 'You're telling my story.' The fifty-year-old woman who stood up and said, 'I am childless—' then stopped mid-sentence, realising that was the first time that she had uttered those words. The black and Asian women who contacted me wanting to talk because they knew that I'd understand. Being interviewed on BBC Radio 4's *Woman's Hour* and for Myleene Klass's *Miscarriage and Me* documentary – I mean, how do they even find me? Oops, could that be self-doubt or my inner bitch speaking? I learnt about my inner bitch, or inner voice, on the Gateway Women's Plan B mentorship programme; the voice that can sometimes feel harsh but is there to guide and protect me. She is always with me and is there to get me to stop and ask myself what I need in that moment.

I'm on this journey because I dared to be vulnerable. I spent a lifetime hiding, as I didn't want anyone to see my inner being. I felt that if they knew me, if they knew what I had done, they wouldn't like me – there's that inner bitch again – but my grief unlocked a door that I then kicked wide open. Everyone is going through something, but we imprison ourselves in shame. We'd be in a better place if we owned our stories, our journeys and what has led us to where we are in that moment, instead of beating ourselves up about it, as that in turn makes us beat each other up. We need to normalise our experiences and remove the self-judgement that keeps us bound in silence.

These moments with other women give me joy, knowing that I am unlocking people's 'stuckness'. Story after story, comment after comment, each positive reaction gave me the strength and courage to keep going. I got to a place where I no longer worried about negative reactions because I wasn't there for those people; I was there for the women who needed to hear me speaking our truth. I am here to give a voice to the voiceless. Finding my voice became my Plan B.

I help women to change the narrative of their own stories when their inner bitches – as well as the external ones – have been telling them that they are wrong, that what they have done is wrong, that they are selfish, that they don't matter. The tough times helped me to go inwards and gain a deeper understanding that allowed me to embrace my light and my shadow, both my own and those I had inherited from previous generations.

In 2019, I spoke at a fertility event about enslaved women not having control over their bodies. Slavery was about ownership. Controlling people's minds and bodies was part of this. Enslaved women didn't have the choice to have a child, when to have a child, or even who to have a child with. Overseers were paid a bonus for each enslaved woman they impregnated. Childless women were seen as worthless, defective stock and punished accordingly. The Alabama physician James Marion Sims conducted his experimental gynaecological surgery exclusively on enslaved black women without anaesthesia because, in his mind, black women didn't feel pain.

Knowing this history helped me to understand the experience I had on my fertility journey. It didn't take away my anger, but it made me more determined to know why I was going through this and to manage the anger I felt towards medical professionals. I received no help when I sat in front of them, begging for relief for my extremely heavy, painful, shitty periods. 'Maybe it's because of your age' was the most I got from them until I presented with severe anaemia, which had to be managed with monthly iron infusions. I was told that the fibroids I had shouldn't cause me any problems with conceiving. It wasn't until I was forty-seven, well after my 'trying for a baby' journey was over, that I was diagnosed with adenomyosis. It felt like no one cared that I couldn't get pregnant when I wanted to.

My infertility wasn't seen as a problem to be solved but as an inconvenience to be tolerated. Everywhere I asked, I found no answers to my questions about why I couldn't get pregnant. It seemed like they were only interested in removing my 'diseased womb' (yes, you heard me; a consultant referred to my adenomyosis that way) to cure my pain.

In her book *Killing the Black Body*, Dorothy Roberts talks about America's history of forced sterilisation, where black women's fertility was seen as a problem to be curbed while white women's infertility was seen as a problem to be cured. It's hard to live with this history, learning that, by and large, a system built on a Eurocentric model wasn't created to help, and isn't interested in helping women who look like me.

In 2016/17, I was offered a hysterectomy because of fibroids (and offered it again following my adenomyosis diagnosis). I looked at the consultant in disbelief, wondering if he was crazy, and then burst into tears. I couldn't believe that this was the only option I was being offered to help with my periods. My womb may not have functioned as expected, but I couldn't see why I needed to lose her. I couldn't understand why having fibroids meant losing my whole womb. It felt like another attack on my femininity, as if not being able to conceive a child wasn't enough.

My therapist helped me to work through the possibility of having a hysterectomy. I realised how angry I was with my body and how hard I found it to like or even look at my stomach. My womb had let me down; she let me get pregnant when I didn't want to and wouldn't when I did. Still, I found it hard to comprehend losing this part of me. I was starting to accept that I wouldn't give birth to my own child, but the absolute finality of this seemed too big to face. One afternoon, I sat down and wrote a letter to say goodbye to my womb. As the words poured onto the paper, my tears poured onto the floor.

I had my hysterectomy in May 2020. I remember sitting in my gown outside the operating theatre when fear suddenly rushed through my body. In that moment it dawned on me that, given all the data around the disparities that black women face in the healthcare system, I might not survive this procedure because I am black.

As much as the quality of my life improved post-surgery, I still have mixed feelings about the procedure. The knowledge that black women are 50 per cent more likely to have a hysterectomy than white women between the ages of eighteen and forty-four, during our most fertile years, brought back all the anger I previously held around the knowledge that black women's fertility is being unconsciously controlled.

Through my childless grief, it dawned on me how much my ancestors had lost through enslavement and how powerful the women who are a part of my history were. I found black childless warriors who built cities in ancient Kemet and led armies to war. Queen Nanny of the Maroons, known by both the Maroons and the British settlers of the eighteenth century as an outstanding military leader, who became a symbol of unity and strength for her people, and Bilikisu Sungbo, a wealthy and accomplished Ijebu widow who was revered by her people, and is mythologised as the Queen of Sheba. Because their choices, dreams and voices were taken away, I realised that I had to fight to reclaim mine. I wanted to give my ancestors and my living sisters our voices back. And so I wear my Wonder Woman knickers and remind myself to speak up because I need to change the narrative. Black women come from a long line of silent sufferers, and I need our generational trauma to be heard and honoured.

It's been a difficult and sometimes scary road, with the realisation that I was afraid to step into my power because of how I would be seen. It often feels like I can't be angry because I might be seen as the 'Angry Black Woman'. Well, this black woman is angry.

- I am angry that my body made the decision not to conceive a child without me.
- I am angry that my fertility journey felt like a fight just to function with some normality on a daily basis.
- I am angry that very few people even want to talk about race – it's the one conversation that gets shut down quicker than you can get past the second letter.
- I am angry at the medical professionals who didn't see a black woman in front of them who needed their help. Black women develop fibroids earlier in life and tend to experience larger and more numerous fibroids that cause more severe symptoms. Nearly a quarter of black women between eighteen and thirty have fibroids compared to about 6 per cent of white women. By age thirty-five, the number increases to 60 per cent. If I know this, then why didn't they? Why didn't this diagnosis occur to them when I came to them with my symptoms?
- I am angry because black women are also at least twice as likely as white women to have their uterus removed through a hysterectomy, a third of which are done during the peak childbearing years between eighteen and forty-four.
- I am angry because black women are diagnosed with endometriosis at older ages than white women. Black women are 49 per cent less likely to get an endometriosis diagnosis compared to white women.

- I am angry because black women have a history of not having autonomy over our bodies, that we lost the freedom to choose when to have a child and who to have a child with – that freedom is still being reclaimed today.
- I am angry because J. Marion Sims performed experiments on enslaved black women to treat vaginal problems without anaesthesia, and because of that, black women are still seen as having a high tolerance of pain.
- I am angry at the unrecognised unconscious conditioning of medical professionals that meant that my pain wasn't believed.
- I am angry that indigenous populations could have their children forcibly removed or stolen from them (between 1910 and 1970) because of the assumption that their lives would be improved if they became part of white society.
- I am angry.

I am a black woman who is ANGRY!

Each painful experience allows me to circle back and go deeper within to understand my hurt and the emotional connection that I have to the pain. I realised that the narrative from our enslaved times was that we mustn't discuss our problems outside of the home so as not to bring shame on our families. The trauma of our enslaved ancestors and enslavers remains with us. My ancestors lived in a time when they couldn't talk. They were punished if they went against the narrative, they remained silent in their pain, and they hid their tears. When their enslavement came to an end, there wasn't a space for them to heal. No one to talk to, no therapy, no one who cared enough to listen. They passed the pain from generation to generation in the language they used to guide us. We need to stop the system from keeping us quiet, from shutting us down. We need to bravely show our cracks, flaws, and all the dark stuff that keeps us enslaved.

Shame for me now is a quiet voice that shows me where I am and where I still need to heal. She shows me my wounds and the pain shows me where I still need to grow whilst looking after my inner child.

The Japanese have a tradition that whenever a plate, jug, vase or cup is broken, it is not discarded as useless but lovingly repaired with gold. Each broken piece is repaired uniquely, and the repair is seen as adding not only to the character and beauty of the original piece but also to its value. I have been broken, and like a kintsugi vase, I have been uniquely repaired. Now I stand proud.


*Yvonne John is an author, speaker, workshop facilitator, activist for childless women of colour and a World Childless Week ambassador. She also works in the NHS.*

# Grief is Not a Competition

*Alice Rose*

'It only took one round of IVF? You're so lucky!'

'Ovulation induction? I've had, like, fifty-four of those.'

'Why did you rush into treatment when it could have just worked naturally?'

In the years since I began supporting people going through variations on a theme – namely, trying to bring home a baby – I have come across the unnecessary one-upmanship, hierarchy, and judgement of other people's experiences of infertility more times than I can say.

It's incredible that while we know so little of anyone's story, we still feel absolutely entitled and fully qualified to cheerfully declare, 'Well, this is what I think about that!' without hearing anything more than the opening head-lines. There is so little room for letting someone share their story.

When my husband Simon and I went through our infer-tility, it was one of the most frustrating seasons of my life. Every time I got my period – or if it was MIA, another regular occurrence – I was grieving. I was grieving every time we had a failed round of fertility treatment, but because that treatment wasn't IVF and because I wasn't experiencing a physical loss, it felt as if I wasn't allowed to be as devastated as I really was.

While there were many times when I did feel supported and held by people in my life, society at large did not get it at all. It was this that felt so isolating and alienating. There was no space for me to share, not without an automatic response of 'It'll happen!' that was suffocating. I felt trapped in a cyclical hellhole of confusion. All I wanted was for someone to say, 'This is so tough for you. You alright, pal? What can I do?'

My husband and I had gone straight into medical intervention when we started trying to bring home our own baby. It's in my nature to get shit done (housekeeping? Not so much. Big life stuff? I am *there*), so as soon as we started to try for a baby, I went to my GP and explained that we would like to have a baby now please and that I had been on the pill for years and years and, oh yes, I've never had a regular menstrual cycle in my life apart from when I'm on fake hormones. And yes, there's been pretty bad acne throughout my teenage and adult life too.

I had vaguely heard of polycystic ovary syndrome (PCOS) but didn't know much about it; only a couple of scary tales some friend at school had shared, like if you had PCOS, it meant you couldn't have a baby.

A healthcare provider had once told me that I might have it, but as I didn't 'present' as a PCOS person – those typical tropes of being heavier and hairier over my body as well as my head, etc. – they thought I was 'probably OK'.

This 'probably OK' meant absolutely bugger all to me. Growing up in the nineties, I didn't have the luxury of

Instagram, with the many brilliant educational accounts and network of peers experiencing the same thing, or the podcasts with hosts who were navigating everything with razor-sharp humour, making their listeners feel normal and relieved it wasn't just them.

All I had was the sketchy school sex ed classes, which explained how straight people had sex and got pregnant (and, of course, how not to) but covered nothing else, absolutely zilch, zero; nothing at all about women's health. There wasn't even the suggestion that we might need to know more about this; why it's completely and utterly integral, not just for fertility awareness but for literally every single other time in a woman's life too.

So, there I was, married a year to my best friend, both of us equally clueless about health. Wonderfully, my GP listened to me and sent me straight off for an ultrasound to see if we could get to the bottom of my irregular cycles, rather than making us struggle on for a year.

I was eventually diagnosed with a medium-sized uterine fibroid and polycystic ovaries – but not the syndrome. This explained my dodgy cycles and crap skin and was a reason to consider going into treatment straight away, as both were likely to have an impact on my fertility.

At no point was it suggested that Simon should be tested to rule out any problems with sperm, which now seems utterly bonkers. Why don't we just do a routine test to check if things are normal before wasting months or possibly years? Makes sense to me, anyway.

I had surgery to remove the fibroid before embarking on ten rounds of ovulation induction. These ten rounds changed me as a person on every level you can imagine. I went through the 'obsessive and neurotic' phase. I went through the 'terrified, sick to my stomach' phase. I went through the WHY DOES NO ONE UNDERSTAND HOW HARD THIS IS? phase and the WHAT THE ACTUAL FUCK IS GOING ON HERE? phase when I received a flurry of correspondence from my NHS clinic cancelling appointments and rearranging them for months in the future when I had already waited what felt like forever.

I went through the angry phase. I went through the 'throw things at my husband because I am changing everything about my existence and you are changing nothing' phase. I went through the 'organic food, alternative therapies, manifesting and vision-boarding and chanting affirmations, manically trying to magic a positive pregnancy into my life' phases too. I thought, *why* don't most of my friends know to tell me what I need to hear? Why does society seem so sure that I'm overreacting when I *feel* like this is deeply, deeply difficult and upsetting? Why are people telling me to 'just adopt'?

I spent hours in hospital with my legs apart, fanny on display, while my internal organs flickered back and forth on a black-and-white screen. I willed my follicles to respond to medication but not too much, of course, for if they respond *too* much we must abandon the cycle. *Abandon.* What a word to use. Abandon it all? All the organic food and injections and stressful rollercoasters on a daily basis with no real confirmation that we will try again and this time it will work?

I went through the phase of sobbing uncontrollably in the nurse's office, the consultant's office, and counsellor's office when I was referred because 'it's clear you're finding this quite stressful'. Yeah, you think?

I went through the 'shooting up like a drug addict in

various public loos across London, sweating when I had too much of an air bubble in the syringe and wondering if I was going to knock the teeny tiny vials over and ruin the entire cycle, or forget a shot or other medication, or somehow not make an appointment because I hadn't marked it in my diary and it clashed with a work commitment' phase.

I went through the 'grateful beyond words to the kindest consultant who stayed late one night when I needed to pick up a prescription for some drugs from the hospital pharmacy and couldn't get there on time' phase.

I went through the 'questioning the clinic and going to allllll the private clinic open days, making notes, collecting promo literature, gathering them all in a big folder and agonising over where to go and when to jump ship from the NHS place, as it wasn't working and I wanted to stop with the ovulation induction because it had been over two years and was completely controlling my life, but they said there were another two rounds I could have and it was a year to wait for IVF' phase.

I went through the 'but what if we pay all this money, which we don't have and will have to borrow and it doesn't work, and we have to pay again and again and maybe again?' phase.

I went through the 'if this doesn't work, what will we do then?' phase.

I went through it all. So did Simon. It wasn't the same as going through multiple rounds of IVF. It wasn't the same physically or emotionally, but does that negate my experience? Because it wasn't IVF, does that invalidate the feelings, emotions and life-changing years? Because I didn't know what it felt like to be pregnant and then lose it?

There is no comparison. There should be no comparison.

No one story makes another one invalid. No story would or could ever take away from the terrible grief of losing pregnancies or spending tens of thousands on unsuccessful IVF. It doesn't mean that grief – yours, mine, theirs – or any of the myriad feelings that come up with it isn't valid.

Some experiences are longer, with more rounds, money spent, and loss endured. This is, of course, true. It seems madness that we would think otherwise. But in my experience, as well as those of people I have helped, there can be an assumption by some that, unless you have been through the 'ultimate' fertility treatment, the 'end of the road' treatment of IVF, then you haven't *really* experienced infertility. Or that, unless you go through any treatment at all, you are not worthy of support or space to share the layered, nuanced avalanche of feelings, fears and anxieties that rise up daily to greet you every morning. Every time you go to the loo and check for blood on the tissue, every time you gear yourself up for another pregnancy announcement because you know it'll make you feel physically sick. That if you haven't had a miscarriage, you don't know grief. That if you haven't spent a shit ton of money on treatment, you can't join the 'infertility sucks' club.

Many people go through infertility without experiencing any treatment at all, either through choice or circumstance. There are so many reasons why someone might not go through IVF.

Ultimately, our journey did end up with IVF. We had one round, which was successful. I had my daughter Matilda in 2016 and her little brother Reggie followed in 2020 from the same batch of embryos. In the end, we went privately for this IVF cycle, and it was a positive and gentle experience. We borrowed the money.

Since I started sharing my story and supporting thousands of women – and men – on Instagram, and later, through my mindset courses, podcast and membership, I have heard it all. Stories of pain, grief, loss, and yet, in amongst it all, treasure, beauty, joy, and something entirely unexpected and wonderful.

I know what it is to hold space for those whose stories differ from mine. I do not compare my own experience. I teach and encourage the members of my community to do the same so that we can gently lift each other up and find positive, self-compassionate ways to navigate the shitshow that is infertility. So that we feel empowered, educated and inspired to continue to see a gentle joy each day in our lives, whatever is going on and however small that joy might be.

Together we work and find hope. Not hope that everyone will have a baby, though I always hope this *is* the case . . . but hope that you will rediscover yourself. You will rediscover yourself and your reason to get up in the morning.

Somewhere in the rounds of treatment, the sobbing, the questioning, the wondering and the fear, I found me again and she was better. More empathetic. More educated and empowered. She was better at holding space, self-compassion, mindfulness and not looking at what other people had and what she wanted.

This revelation led me to seek out others going through infertility or any difficult road to parenthood and let them know there was a way to find a sort of gentle peace with the whole thing. They wouldn't feel this all day, every day, no no. It's just that it was available with the proper support and deeply compassionate understanding from people who got it.

I wanted them to know that, no, it was not their fault they were finding it overwhelming and that yes, people do make infuriating comments and no, it didn't mean they weren't experiencing something really hard.

That's what I need to say, time and again. Your story is valid. It isn't your fault. None of it is your fault. And there is hope. When we're listened to, heard, seen and held, there is hope for beauty, joy and self-compassionate living, whatever else is going on in life.

So try not to compare my story with others you might read about. Try not to compare your own. Try to stay absolutely focused on your own experience and know that there are spaces where you will be heard and held and seen and that those people there will meet you exactly where you're at.

*Alice Rose is a transformation coach, and the creator of the Fertility Life Raft community and the Think! What Not To Say campaign against infertility stigma.*

# 'Other People' Problems

*Gemma Stone*

I was at a baby shower the other day. My friend is pregnant as hell, and they threw a little baby-themed barbecue with a handful of games like 'guess the baby-food flavour'. My partner and I were named godparents and invited to become legal guardians. Of course, we said yes! I'm so happy for them and, being as close as we are, hell yes am I down to help raise this child in whatever way is required of me. A joyously positive reaction I doubt I would've had a few years ago.

That's because I wasn't in as good a place as I am today with regards to my general mental health, and specifically on the topic of motherhood. I've always wanted kids. I think so, anyway. It's hard to really tell. What I know for certain is that I have expressed deep sadness about my inability to have my own biological children. You know those times when you look wistfully off into the distance and start to daydream about your future? Mine have often involved helping to raise a family with my partner, only for big dark clouds to roll in over the scene as the reality of my situation starts to seep into the idealised fantasy.

The reality is that I will probably never be able to have the same experience as my friend. I will never be pregnant; I will never develop a cute little waddle or stand around rubbing my tummy and shouting at people to come feel it kick. I will never give birth to my own child or, indeed, have my own child at all. This is a reality that many women experience for many different reasons. For me it's because I'm a transgender woman and – right now? – I am OK with this.

Not that there aren't attempts being made to change this for all women, including us transgender ones. There obviously are, more than you'd think, in fact. One of the headlines I read a few years ago, in 2017, was the *Independent*'s 'Trans women could get pregnant "tomorrow", fertility professor claims', an article I shared around a lot because of my excitement at the prospect. Another paper from 2019 titled 'Uterine transplantation in transgender women' remarks on using a technique developed in 2014 for cisgender women that had successfully resulted in a dozen or so live births in Sweden. Even as recently as May 2022, there were reports in *Business Insider*, the *Daily Mail* and on UNILAD about Dr Narendra Kaushik, in India, proposing to attempt the technique for transgender women and calling it 'the future' for us.

A few years ago, I'd have been desperate to know more. I'd have been researching this doctor, looking through papers about the transplant and finding expert opinions on its viability in trans women. Maybe even booking my own trip out to New Delhi! I've only ever been as far as Ibiza before, but if this option had been on the table a few years sooner, I don't think there is a lot that could have stopped me scraping together the cash to afford the procedure, trip, and recovery time. I felt desperate to be able to give birth and it's probably important to explore why.

The first thing you'll be told as a transgender woman is that you can't possibly be a real woman because a real woman is a woman that can give birth. Every transphobe has their own flavour of this rhetoric: some will say 'only women have a cervix' or that because trans women have never had to fear unwanted pregnancies, experienced the onset of periods, or had to explain ourselves to a lady in Boots when trying to get the morning-after pill, we simply can't be women. Of course, they ignore the many cis women for whom these experiences also don't apply. The framing is that trans women's lives and the average cis woman's life are fundamentally too different to be described by the same word: woman. But really it all boils down to the same thing: the belief that a woman is supposed to be able to have babies.

The worst example of this sent my way in my almost-decade of writing on trans issues came on Twitter in 2018. A user who was proud enough of her own motherhood to heavily adorn her profile in references to it wrote to me, 'Do you love the fact that you'll never have a body that actually does anything? I do. I'm so happy you cut up your body and can't have kids now.' I had it saved on my phone as a screenshot – not that I needed to. I remembered those words for a long time. They cut pretty deep back then.

This rhetoric is so entrenched that people from politicians to Olympic athletes and even lifelong feminist campaigners not only acknowledge it but actively reinforce it. It was even the subject of a TV advert for sanitary products in 2012, for Australian brand Libra, in which a cis woman and a trans woman do a little bit of feminine competition in a bathroom mirror, one-upping each other over hairstyles and tit sizes. It ends with the cis woman 'winning' by pulling a tampon out of her bag to prove she is the most woman-est. Libra Tampons later pulled the campaign and apologised after complaints about how this was insensitive to both trans and cis women.

Even further, many people who don't believe trans women can really be women because we can't give birth have mocked the idea that we would even want to. In her 1999 book *The Whole Woman*, Germaine Greer suggested that 'if uterus-and-ovaries transplants were made mandatory for wannabe women they would disappear overnight'. Others have scraped the bottom of the horrific barrel to tweet their hope that such uterine transplants would spread through our bodies like 'a thousand cancers',* causing a gruesome death. Complete with an evil grin, no less!

Suffice to say, this is not an easy thing to have to navigate. It wasn't until recently that I had any idea whether the desperation I felt came from within me, or if it was more informed by social pressure to conform to a society's transphobic and misogynist standards of what a woman should be. If I'm honest, I still don't really know, but I've found it helps to pick an answer, wear it around a little, and see how it fits.

The one I've picked is working out pretty OK and I feel good about it. Good enough not to be overwhelmingly sad whilst in the vicinity of baby stuff, anyway. My answer is that no one is born destined for any kind of parenthood. No one is born wanting to menstruate or have a functional uterus. The expectation placed on all women – including women like me – is that being a good woman means giving birth to a baby, so we learn to feel bad when we can't, or have it held against us

---

* @FairPlayForWomen on Twitter, 2018 www.pinknews.co.uk/2018/10/12/fair-play-for-women-tweets-1000-cancers/)

if we don't want to. If it's something we learned, it's something we can work to unlearn. We can stop passing it to the next generation of women and furthering that cycle of hurt.

How did I come to this conclusion? The short answer is other people. The long answer is a journey through those swamps of transphobia, which, for all its faults, has helped shape me into a much stronger woman than I was before I attempted to engage with it. Not because of the transphobia itself, dear Lorde no. The psychic damage I have taken from engaging with transphobia, especially the vapid sock-puppet accounts and anti-trans 'activism' on social media, is immeasurable. You should not put yourself through that. The benefit, for me at least, has come from the little pockets of resistance that have popped up around it.

It's through these beautiful chunks of solidarity from people of all stripes, and family units of all configurations, that I've come to figure myself out more and altogether have a better time of life. Transphobes told me what a woman *should* be, but glorious queers and allies showed me that a woman *can* be anything she damn well pleases. They tore down the rigid structures that defined people like me out of having a family or being a mother and showed me how to build a better idea in its place. One that doesn't outright punish or discard you for not fitting in, instead opting to just make space for you.

Most impressive of all is that I don't think they were even trying to tear those structures down. They just did it by existing. Passively, even. I've become friends with a lot of different parents, some foster parents, some step-parents, some adoptive parents, some parents that are found family. I've also become friends with a lot of different women who all have their own unique stories and have taught me how to expand my view of womanhood. A woman doesn't have to be a mother, but she can if she wants to be. She doesn't have to give birth to her own child to be a mother, but she can if she wants to. She doesn't have to call herself a mother even if she does give birth, but she can if she wants to.

Just existing near these people, learning about them, taking part in their lives and letting them into mine has changed my outlook on everything. I've never felt more me or happier than I do today, and I owe a lot of that to those around me for immersing me in love and support.

I don't know the source of the desperation I felt to be a birth mother. I don't think I'll ever be able to truly know if it came from me or from society – it won't become apparent until those societal norms no longer exist. I don't even know if my feelings about wanting to be a mother will ever fully go away, but I don't need to anymore. I've found a much greater answer to the problem I was facing, and that answer brings me so much peace, joy and security.

I know that if and when I choose to be a mother, I'll be an absolutely badass one. It won't make a bit of difference whether I become a mother through fostering, adoption, or some future technique to allow transgender women to get pregnant. I am not missing out on anything by having a different experience of motherhood from someone else. I also know that, even if I choose not to be a mother, I am still a kick-ass woman. I know that the fact I can't give birth is irrelevant to the equation. I love who I am and the only thing I have to be ashamed of letting people like that Twitter user and their hateful, mean-spirited nonsense get to me. A mistake I won't be making again any time soon!

That's why I jumped at the opportunity to be part of this book. Resources like this are so important because, as the title says, no one talks about this stuff. I struggled with my feelings fairly quietly and on my own for so long. It's only through passively hearing of other people in similar situations and their perspectives that I've been able to turn a source of deep discomfort into something really quite positive and uplifting, actually.

I want to be part of that for someone else: I want to make an active effort to help others find the peace from these societal norms that I now enjoy. I hope that I, and the other writers here, have helped you achieve that.

*Gemma Stone is a freelance writer and the co-founder of Trans Writes (transwrites.world), a transgender-led platform that seeks out and publishes writings exclusively from transgender creators.*

# Choice

# Elodie

*Hilary Freeman*

'Why should a dog, a horse, a rat have life,
And thou no breath at all? Oh, thoult come no more,
Never, never, never, never, never.
Pray you, undo this button. Thank you, sir.
Do you see this? Look on her. Look, her lips.'

Shakespeare, *King Lear*, Act 5, Scene 3

At 11.51 p.m. on Wednesday, 26 September 2012, I gave birth to my first child, a daughter named Elodie. She had died on Monday afternoon; oddly, I don't recall the precise hour. She was twenty-three weeks and six days gestation.

This is not the story of a stillbirth, although it shares some painful similarities. In the darkest days following Elodie's death, I'm ashamed to say that I actually envied those who experience that terrible class of baby loss. My daughter's death was neither accident nor tragedy: it was a deliberate act, and one which I consented to. Medical terminology calls what I did feticide. It is also known as a termination for medical reasons (TFMR), which is no less clinical-sounding, but perhaps less emotive.

I am only too aware that there are people – I hope nobody reading this book – who would have me condemned or imprisoned for my actions. I know this because several of them sent me unsolicited emails and social media messages when I first talked about what happened, in a newspaper article, soon afterwards. For some unknown, masochistic reason, I have kept these messages, the ones begging me to repent or damning me to hell. The more I read them, the less they sting.

I will tell you the how first. The why will come later. Forget any propaganda images you may have seen regarding TMFR. You can't have a surgical abortion late on in pregnancy – at least, not on the NHS. Neither can you have a Caesarean. You must go through a full labour and give birth, and, before you do this, doctors prefer to make sure that there's no chance your baby will be born alive.

Elodie died at the steady hands of an obstetrician, while I lay still on an examination table in the Fetal Medicine Unit at University College Hospital in London. Mickaël, my then boyfriend, now civil partner, held my hand as potassium chloride was injected into her heart. This is the same drug used in execution by lethal injection in several US states (ironically, in some of the same states where TFMR is now illegal).

I wasn't allowed to watch my daughter die, even though I felt strangely compelled to; the ultrasound screen in front of me was switched off. So, I closed my eyes and cried silently until it was done, feeling Elodie's kicks right until the end.

For the next twenty minutes, an eternity, I had to remain there while the doctors did more tests and scans to be certain her heart was no longer beating. The mood in the room was sombre, respectful. Nobody spoke; even my tendency to make nervous small talk in dark situations was quelled. On the other side of the curtain lay another sobbing woman, whose face I never saw. I overheard the doctors telling her that her scan showed her baby had a brain problem, and I remember feeling irrationally jealous because at least her baby was still alive.

Afterwards, I was taken into another room and given a drug to soften my cervix in preparation for birth. As the nurse handed the tablet over, I fumbled it, all fingers and thumbs, and watched in horror as it dropped, rolled across the floor and came to rest under a desk. With a shriek, the nurse went chasing after it, launching herself on to the floor on all fours to retrieve it. There aren't many moments of light relief in my story, but this was pure slapstick, and extreme emotions can lead to inappropriate reactions. I found myself laughing hysterically at the ridiculousness of the situation and at the black humour in it. Unfortunately, the nurse didn't see the funny side: 'This is a controlled drug!' she cried, chastising me, before dusting it off and handing it to me with a cup of water, making sure I swallowed it in front of her.

For the two days between Elodie's death and her birth – it still strikes me how counterintuitive it is to put those words in that illogical order – I carried her corpse inside me, attempting some semblance of normality. I remember walking around Selfridges, looking at the new winter clothes which I knew would soon fit again, but shouldn't. Only a few weeks earlier I'd been buying maternity dresses. There were moments in which I was convinced I could feel Elodie kicking me; phantom kicks, like the pain from an amputated limb.

Nothing was supposed to happen until I was induced on

Wednesday afternoon, but on Tuesday night I began to suffer painful cramps. By Wednesday morning I was bleeding heavily and having contractions. The hospital told us to come straight in. We took a taxi. 'I'm having a baby,' I said to the driver, pointlessly. 'That's nice,' he replied, casting his eyes dubiously over my compact, six-month bump, perhaps anxious that my waters might break and leave a mess on his leatherette seats.

On arrival, Mickaël and I were put in a side room on the labour ward, away from the other mothers and out of earshot of their crying, living babies. It was called the Butterfly Room and decorated as such, as if that would somehow make the conveyor belt of labouring mothers, dead babies and grieving parents within less unpleasant.

I'm not going to sugarcoat the details, but I will spare you some of the more visceral ones. Giving birth to Elodie was traumatic and extremely painful. I was given morphine, which did nothing for my pain, but did make me projectile vomit the cheese sandwich from the vending machine which I'd forced down at lunchtime and led me to hallucinate giant teddy bears and old men at the end of the bed. The anaesthetist didn't come, despite being called several times, so I couldn't have the promised epidural and relied on gas and air. My malformed placenta 'abrupted' – detached from my womb – leading to the loss of almost two litres of blood. Twelve hours later, I was still so weak that I collapsed in the shower and had to be carried out naked in a wheelchair.

But here's that masochistic tendency again: in a way, I felt I deserved all this as punishment for taking my baby's life. This is a reaction I'm told is not unusual among women in my situation.

Elodie was 'born sleeping' – the euphemism people find

most palatable – weighing just over a pound. She was tiny but perfect, with her father's Cupid's-bow lips and my hands. She looked so peaceful that seeing her took away my fear of death, at least in the short term.

The midwives cleaned and dressed her in a babygro and a little woolly hat before they brought her back to us. We held her and talked to her, had photos taken with her, and admired her tiny fingers and fingernails, just as you would any newborn. And for a while I felt euphoric – one of nature's cruel hormonal tricks – until I realised that she was growing ice cold, and it hit me that she would never be warm again.

I saw Elodie just twice more. Later that night, I woke up shivering with cold and shock, opened my eyes and caught sight of the empty cot, which had been left next to my bed. Struck by the reality of what had happened, I became hysterical and could only be comforted when she was brought back to me to hold.

The last time was the next morning, just before we left the hospital. Despite being kept in a cold room, by now her paper-thin skin had begun to whiten and wrinkle, and her mouth was lolling open. We knew then that it was time to say goodbye.

Elodie was cremated at Golders Green Crematorium the following week, in a funeral service arranged by the hospital's charity. Two months later, I travelled to Nice, France, where Mickaël lived at the time, and where Elodie had been conceived. We scattered her ashes on a secluded cove beach, watching as the wind carried her out to sea.

Elodie was a very much wanted baby. To our surprise, I fell pregnant the very first week we started trying, a month shy of my forty-first birthday. Even though Mickaël and I were then in a long-distance relationship, and I was in the midst of a complicated and nasty divorce, we were naively optimistic that the logistics would work out. I'd wanted a baby for years; my ex-husband hadn't.

The first time I knew something might be wrong was at eight weeks, when a scan showed that my embryo and gestational sac were too small. I was warned I might miscarry at any moment. But, against all odds, my embryo kept on growing and her heart kept on beating. Then, at twelve weeks, routine blood tests showed markers for Down's syndrome. I underwent a screening procedure called a chorionic villus sampling (CVS), in which cells are taken from the placenta and tested for chromosome problems. It was unsuccessful: my placenta was too thick and strangely textured. The consultant obstetrician said he had never seen a placenta like it.

At sixteen weeks, a second CVS revealed that my baby didn't have Down's, or the other common chromosome conditions. The consultant concluded that the problem lay solely with my weird placenta, which wasn't functioning properly. I was warned it could fail at any time and that my baby might not make it. If she did, she would be very small and premature.

Termination was an option, the consultant said. At that stage, I refused. How could I kill a wanted baby, who might survive and be fine? By now I knew I was carrying a girl, whom we'd named Elodie, and I already thought of her as a little person. But worse news was to come. Three weeks later, by which time I had started to feel her move inside me, I received a shocking phone call. Trisomy 2 cells, which are indicators of a potential chromosome problem, had been found in my second CVS placental sample. I would need an amniocentesis to see if the baby was also affected. For a third time, a needle was passed through my abdomen into my womb to collect my baby's cells. Each time this happened, I risked miscarriage. Yet each time, Elodie survived and continued to grow.

I was twenty-two weeks pregnant when I finally learned the reason for her growth restriction and my placental issues. The full amniocentesis results showed that she had a chromosome condition called trisomy 2 mosaicism (an extra copy of chromosome 2), which is so rare that there are only a handful of children known to be living with it in the world. Chromosome 2 is fundamental to human life, meaning that, usually, any problem with it causes spontaneous early miscarriage. But, in a tiny handful of pregnancies, like mine with Elodie, the foetus continues to develop. Nobody knows why. Nature, I learned, does not always have a plan. It can be random and cruel.

Each of the surviving children I read about in medical papers were living with severe, but different, disabilities: among them brain damage, feeding problems, heart and kidney problems, and physical deformities. I was warned that, if I chose to continue with my pregnancy, it was very likely that Elodie would die, either before birth or shortly afterwards. The only positive news was that this was something so rare and unrelated to my age that, if I tried for another baby, it could never happen again.

The doctors all made it clear that they thought a termination was for the best, but the decision about what to do was mine, and mine alone. There was no rush; the twenty-four-week legal time limit didn't apply in cases like mine. Mickaël said he'd be supportive of whatever I chose, but he was also clear that it wouldn't be fair to let our baby suffer.

When I asked him if he'd be able to cope with a severely disabled child, he was very honest. 'I really don't know,' he said. How can anyone know?

For days after the diagnosis, I prayed I would miscarry, that nature would make the decision for me. But nature, as I said earlier, is cruel. My belly kept expanding and Elodie kept kicking. Each kick felt like a plea. There is a biological instinct to protect the being growing inside you; everything from your hormones to your immune system is primed to do so. You start to convince yourself that the doctors might be wrong and that, even if they aren't, it doesn't matter what problems your baby may have because you will love her anyway.

In the end, two people persuaded me that my only option was to terminate. The first was a consultant geneticist at Great Ormond Street Hospital who made it very clear that if I continued with my pregnancy, Elodie's life would be, to borrow from Thomas Hobbes, 'nasty, brutish and short'. For however long she survived, she would suffer physically and emotionally. He assured me that if I were to terminate my pregnancy, she would not feel anything and her death would be instant. On the other hand, being born alive through a delivery would cause her great trauma.

The second was an old friend, who had severely disabled twins, born very prematurely. She reminded me how much her children have suffered, and how much the rest of the family has suffered, too. She said that as a good mother, I could only make one decision for my baby: to end her life to prevent her suffering.

Caught between a rock and a hard place, I chose the 'least worst' option.

In the days leading up to the feticide, it felt as if Elodie was on death row. I started planning for her funeral, choosing the music and the readings, even though she was still kicking inside me. I also had to choose the outfit she would wear in her coffin, which I bought from a specialist website selling clothes for premature and stillborn babies. I bought a blanket too, and three miniature teddy bears: one for Mickaël, one for me, and one for Elodie.

It was all such a mindfuck that I found myself wondering if she somehow sensed what I was planning. Sometimes, I would stroke my belly and tell her I was sorry. And sometimes, even though I'm an atheist, I prayed for her forgiveness.

You know the rest.

A week before Elodie's death and birth, I went with a friend to see *King Lear* at the Almeida Theatre in Islington. In retrospect, it was a foolish choice of play, but it starred Jonathan Pryce, it was a hot ticket, and I didn't think it through. For those who don't know Shakespeare, it's the tragedy of a foolish and vain old king who divides his kingdom between his three daughters, realising too late that he has wronged and rejected the one who truly loved him. In his last speech, after she has been executed as a result of his actions, he says: 'Look on her, look, her lips / Look there, look there!' Then, mad with grief, he dies too. It's a play about many things – the loss of hope and innocence, greed, and politics – but for me, just days away from losing my own beloved daughter, it was unbearable to watch. As the rest of the audience clapped, I bawled. And a week later, when I looked at Elodie's lips, I couldn't help but be reminded of those lines again.

The history of literature is full of tales of child loss and child killing. In the Bible, when God wanted to punish the

Egyptians, he saved the most terrible plague for last: the deaths of the firstborn. (I once cried watching the musical *The Prince of Egypt* too; my grief doesn't only have highbrow taste.) Greek mythology contains countless examples of mortals and gods killing their own and other people's children, often in revenge. Why? Because losing a child is supposed to be the worst experience that can befall a person; because it goes against the natural order of things.

But, remember that nature gets it wrong sometimes. It fucks up. Animals that give birth to sickly young who won't survive reject, or even kill and eat them. Maybe, you could argue, I did the most natural thing in the world.

Whenever I hear that someone has murdered a child, my reaction – like everyone else's – is horror. But then a dreadful thought strikes me: I did just that; I killed my own child too. And, while I know it's not ethically or morally the same – that I am not a murderer, that I did the right thing for the right reasons – sometimes it feels like it is.

Let me be very clear here: despite the emotive language that I'm using, I am 100 per cent pro-choice. I believe every woman should have the right to have an abortion for whatever reason motivates her. I do not expect her to feel any guilt or regret.

Nevertheless, I feel there is a vast difference between the abortion of an unwanted and a wanted baby. What I experienced seems to me to be a kind of halfway house between abortion and stillbirth. I feel little in common with the woman who gets accidentally pregnant and takes an abortion pill, or who has an early surgical procedure, painful as those decisions are to make. Neither can I relate to the woman who suffers the terrible tragedy of unexplained stillbirth.

The psychological and emotional impact of taking the decision to end the life of your much-wanted child is not easily explainable. There is a complex tangle of grief and guilt, the rational wrestling endlessly with the emotional. I haven't had any counselling, although perhaps it would have been helpful early on; the NHS funding was not available at the time I requested it. Instead, I have coped with my grief in the only way I know how: by talking, by writing, by keeping Elodie alive in words. I have been relentlessly, some would say annoyingly, open because I know that the more you talk about something, the less power it has to hurt or shame you. A wonderful, unintended consequence of this openness is the friendships it has brought me with other women, women who have suffered similar losses, who contacted me after hearing my story. Knowing that my words helped them has brought me comfort too.

Eleven years on, I do not think about Elodie all the time as I once did, but I am still grieving. I now realise that I always will be. It is not a normal type of bereavement. I have no happy memories to cling to, just traumatic ones. I can imagine what might have been, but it will never be a reality. I am mourning a potential life, rather than a lived one, a being who will always be both a stranger and a part of me.

It's also a lonely grief. No one else met Elodie, save Mickaël and the two midwives who were with me at her birth. Mickaël is sad too, of course, but he did not grow her inside his body or feel her kick; he did not give birth to her.

Women have only been making decisions like the one I had to make for the past thirty years or so, since scanning and screening techniques became good enough to allow doctors to diagnose serious conditions in utero. And there really aren't very many of us. Only around 500 women each year in the UK have a termination after twenty-two weeks under Ground E, the legal clause in abortion legislation allowing TFMR.

At the turn of the twenty-first century, TFMR was available to women in approximately 39 per cent of the countries in the world. But globally, our abortion rights are under attack, with anti-abortion rhetoric growing louder. In the ten years since I had Elodie, TFMR has become illegal in several US states, as well as in Poland. Women facing decisions like mine will have a choice between a dangerous backstreet abortion, or travelling abroad for help, both adding to the trauma and making it financially impossible for many.

At the same time, here in the UK there is a growing campaign calling for an end to late-term (after twenty-four weeks) abortion in cases of severe disability, on the grounds of discrimination. While I appreciate that many people with Down's syndrome are now able to live full and rewarding lives thanks to medical developments (although levels of disability vary), that is not the case for all of those born with severe disabilities. Sometimes it is not clear cut whether a condition will prove fatal, or for how long someone with it might live. Severe disabilities are often not diagnosed until late on in a pregnancy, even in the weeks leading up to birth. Reducing the abortion time limit in cases of foetal abnormality would actually achieve the opposite of its desired effect, by forcing women to rush a decision before they are armed with the full facts.

When I meet people who have severely disabled children, I sometimes feel guilty and apologetic, as if what I chose is an affront to their very existence. I have to remind myself that I didn't choose to end Elodie's life because I thought it would have less value than a healthy baby's but because I wanted to spare her pain and suffering and an almost certain early death. I believe every woman should have the right to make her own choice.

In June 2015, almost three years after I 'lost' Elodie, and following two miscarriages, I gave birth to another daughter whom we named Sidonie. She is now a happy, healthy, beautiful and bright eight-year-old.

Sidonie would dearly love a sibling. She knows she had an older sister named Elodie, who was very sick and who died before she was born, although she doesn't yet know how or why. One day, she will learn that I chose to end her sister's life, and I am braced for the inevitable question: 'Would you have killed me too, if I had been sick like her?'

How can I even begin to answer that?

Every year on Elodie's birthday, we light a candle in her memory. And on 1 September 2020, in the midst of the pandemic, my little family packed up our London flat and moved onto a houseboat in Limehouse Marina. We christened our brand-new wide-beam barge *Elodie* in tribute to our late daughter, and had her name engraved in gold letters on her stern. Now she will always sail with us.

*Hilary Freeman is a journalist, novelist and advice columnist.*

# Flashbacks and Tricycles: Chosen Childlessness and Trauma Disorders

*Quinn Clark*

As a teenager, I worked in a children's science museum. What a job! I spent my days in a vibrant educational playground, dressing up in silly costumes and supporting children in the development of their scientific knowledge. It was impossible not to develop a joy for working with kids; innovative, innately artistic individuals whose love for creation hasn't yet been marred by adults telling them what kind of work is 'good' or 'bad'.

Now, as a twenty-something in a creative industry, it's hard not to envy children and their ability to enjoy making art with no strings attached. I reckon we could all stand to learn a thing or two from children in this regard. Perhaps they can be a touch infuriating from time to time – such as when they decide to cut up and paint a bunch of your shirts to make a Pokémon costume, like I did at that age – but they're still fascinating human beings. They must be, or else we wouldn't keep having them!

If only having children were an easy task. Physical and financial issues are just two of the prominent obstacles facing potential parents. Many are unable to become pregnant, carry a child to term, or give birth, whilst countless others lack the money and job security needed to provide a child with a safe, healthy upbringing. The reasons for childlessness are complex and personal, and we would do well not to pressure those around us into explaining why they don't have children.

Well, what if you *could* have kids but you don't want to?

Here's the thing: I hit puberty when I was seven. 'Precocious puberty' is a condition where puberty happens well before the expected age. For me, this meant at six I was already developing breasts and acne. I was seven when I got my first period, and I was biologically capable of having children years before I was even a teenager.

I feel this puberty context is important, even though I don't want to share too much about this part of my life. Being a trauma survivor is a part of my identity I've always been candid about, and much of my work as an author, poet and creative writing facilitator is informed by those experiences. However, the specifics of my trauma are not relevant to this conversation. All you need to know is the following: I emerged from my teenage years with a less-than-stellar relationship with my parents and a fabulous diagnosis of complex post-traumatic stress disorder (CPTSD).

Don't worry too much about the differences between PTSD and CPTSD yet. First, I'd like to talk about what trauma is. When we refer to trauma, we're usually talking about traumatic events and our responses to them. A traumatic event is any event that causes significant physical, psychological or emotional harm. This could be anything from bullying, to surviving a car crash or being a victim of human trafficking. There is no one-size-fits-all description. What is traumatic to one person may not be to another, and it is important not to draw comparisons or try to stake claims about 'who had it worse'. Although the duration and severity of symptoms may differ between survivors, everyone with trauma deserves to feel validated, and should never have their experiences diminished.

At eighteen years old and standing at only four feet ten inches – precocious puberty can stunt your growth – I was scarcely taller than any of the under-tens pouring in to play with our plasma globe. But a few days passed and interacting with the kids became easier. It turns out that children respond well to creative encouragement and silly puns, and I am nothing if not armed with both!

One day, I was tasked with overseeing a craft station. Kids could come in and make their own musical shakers out of cardboard, beads and fabric. Everything was going well, and the kids were having a great time. But, out of the corner of my eye, I noticed one child sequestering himself from the others who was very much not making a musical shaker. Instead, he had cut, threaded and glued a variety of tubes, string and pom-poms into some kind of elaborate walkie-talkie system, straight out of a Rube Goldberg machine. Intrigued, I went over:

'What are you making?'

The kid looked up with bright eyes. 'Spy phones!'

Cue this brilliant little child spending the next twenty minutes enthusiastically giving a play-by-play account of an elaborate fictional universe he had created: a high-octane spy thriller full of betrayal, espionage and novel technology. I was enthralled. The amount of time and effort this kid poured into his world was equal parts astonishing and humbling, and I did my best to let him know exactly that. He responded with a smile so brilliant I couldn't help but grin right back. And for a moment, a little thought crept into the back of my mind:

*Maybe I do want to have kids.*

Then his mother came over.

'Thanks for taking the time to indulge him,' she confided in me with a shy smile. 'He's so creative, I don't always know what to say.'

I returned the smile, thanked her and her son for coming, and told the kid to send me a copy of his book when he's famous. I held that smile in a static, frozen position, all while watching their slowly retreating backs until they made their way out of the museum.

And then I let my supervisor know I was popping to the loo, locked myself in a toilet stall, and had a full-blown, trembling panic attack.

I couldn't tell you what it was that triggered me that day. Perhaps the mother's kindness reminded me of the lack of stability I had during my younger years. Maybe the kid feeling comfortable enough to be outspoken and excited about his passions left me off-kilter, remembering how dangerous that was for me as a neurodivergent child. That's the thing about trauma: even if you have a clear, pinpointable traumatic event in your past, the trauma itself gets stored in your brain as a jumble of sensations and emotions. It's not always as straightforward as the sound of a firework reminding a veteran of gunshots.

The mechanisms of trauma are simple. When we experience something significantly distressing, our brain and body work to help us survive the traumatic event. You may have heard of 'fight, flight or freeze', an uncontrollable, physiological response that activates when we are confronted with a threat. A flood of chemicals and hormones kicks your body into action, trying to neutralise, get you away from, or even *bore* the threat into leaving you alone. It's a survival method born from evolution and something that helps us overpower, outrun and deceive predators. Pretty amazing, when you think about it.

However, this response comes with a price. Because our brains are so focused on surviving the traumatic events, something funny happens to the way memories of the events are stored. The science is much more complicated than I'm qualified to share, but a good way to think of it is that the trauma memories 'sit on top' of your brain in fragments. They aren't filed away properly the way your other memories are.

For instance, let's say you cried the first time you saw a sad film, an emotionally reactive moment, but not necessarily a traumatic one. Chances are, if you remember that moment, you won't burst into tears. Trauma memories are different because, when activated, the memory replays in your brain *as if it is happening for the first time.*

Earlier I used the word 'triggered', and *triggers* are another commonly misunderstood aspect of the traumatised experience. They go hand in hand with *flashbacks*: the reliving of a moment from the past through images, sounds and other fractured pieces of memory, including scents, tactile sensations and even emotions. A trigger is something that sets off a flashback. Triggers can be random: a turn of phrase, an old song, or even the taste of a certain food. The jumbled, broken way trauma memories get stored (because your brain was far too focused on keeping you alive to process the memory in full) means that two people with similar trauma can have vastly different triggers.

I used to break out in cold sweats having dinner with my ex-partner's parents. Walking past a playground would make me completely tune out, and I'd wind up back home twenty minutes later with no recollection of how I got there. Even hearing a parent compliment their child – like the mother at the science museum – caused an awful, adverse reaction because even thinking about raising a family is, for me and many others, inexorably traumatic. Having PTSD turns the world into a metaphorical minefield. You never know what might trigger a flashback, turning on that fight, flight or freeze response and leaving you terrified, shaking and sick.

It's complicated. I love kids: I think they're fantastic, I enjoy being around them, and I believe they should be protected, nurtured and encouraged at every turn. But because of my condition, I know that I am unable to provide a safe space for a child to grow and mature. People often think of PTSD as a temporary condition or something that only affects veterans. They hold in their heads the idea of a grizzled, silent war hero who has suffered greatly, but talks about the horrors they've seen as glorious. The truth is that trauma survivors come in a variety of shapes and sizes, and we need to do better at acknowledging diversity in what survivors look like and how we behave.

Let's get this out of the way: trauma disorders cannot be cured by internalising 'mind over matter', and there is no threshold for what is traumatic. In fact, the pervasive idea that mind and body are somehow separate is a great barrier to those seeking help for trauma. The physical symptoms of

PTSD – hyperventilation, nausea/vomiting, trembling, etc. – are a direct result of our nervous system being flooded with those aforementioned chemicals, trying to keep us alive in the face of a threat. PTSD is like a faulty alarm system. For those with trauma, there was a time when we needed the sensitivity of our internal alarms to be high to protect us from danger – we needed to be on guard to stay alive. But it is when we are free from the danger that these reactive, biological behaviours turn disordered, and their frequency and severity become harmful.

It may seem counterintuitive, but for myself and many survivors it is the mundane parts of life that are the hardest – and that is exactly why, at this time of writing, I cannot raise a kid safely. It's not any survivor's fault that we perceive danger where it may not exist; it's simply a consequence of our physiology. When people have extended or inescapable trauma – for instance, being in a war zone or living with someone abusive – our nervous systems become exhausted and highly strung after working overtime to protect us when needed. This specific symptom of PTSD is called *hypervigilance*, and it involves being constantly on guard for threats. Hypervigilance is a state that is entered unconsciously; it causes our brains to strain to hear sounds we may otherwise miss, or to see things out of the corner of our eye that may pose a threat. It's difficult to truly express how much hypervigilance takes its toll on a body, but it wipes you out. Have you ever been told to stop tensing your jaw because it's giving you pain? There's your answer to the migraines, irritable bowels, tingling extremities, overactive bladders and nausea common with trauma survivors, amongst other ailments: our bodies respond with sickness because they're overwrought.

Combined with the unpredictable nature of triggers, hyper-vigilance makes it all too easy for a trauma survivor to become overwhelmed. Imagine that everything is twenty times louder than it sounds to everyone else, and small movements look like large, sweeping attacks. Add that to neurodivergence and pre-existing conditions, which include sensory overload (having already heightened senses), and suddenly it doesn't seem so strange that an innocuous situation can send us into a spiral. As an autistic person with a trauma disorder, even existing in my own home – a relatively stable, relaxed environment – can be impossible some days. While there are plenty of parents with trauma who can navigate their hypervigilance whilst successfully raising a child, this is not something I am capable of – and that is not a cause for shame.

Hypervigilance doesn't exist in a vacuum, either. The human brain is accomplished at shoving things down for later, assuming there will be a better, safer point to process something terrible. When we're exposed to repeated, extreme trauma, this adaptation can cause some unusual problems.

*Dissociation* is a mental disconnect from your surroundings, self and/or personality. Everyone dissociates to some degree, such as when you zone out while driving or daydream during a meeting, but dissociation due to trauma is for a specific purpose. When trauma memories are activated, instead of experiencing all those dreadful, fragmented bits of trauma all at once, sometimes trauma survivors enter a dissociative state. This state is involuntary and is characterised by a *flat affect* (not exhibiting one's emotions and speaking in a mono-tone) and unusual sensory experiences. It may seem as though you can't feel your arms or legs, like you're looking through a fishbowl, or even like everyone around you is flat and made of cardboard. Think of it like turning off background programs on a computer when you're rendering a big file – your brain has decided to remove the excess sensation so you can continue functioning.

Understandably, for those who have severe and complex trauma, dissociative states can feel preferable to experiencing the physical and mental effects of processing traumatic memories. This is why some individuals with trauma develop dissociative disorders. These disorders involve dissociation happening so frequently or to such an intense degree that they disrupt typical processes of memory, function and identity. Those with dissociative disorders may disconnect from reality or struggle to recall specific periods of their lives. I am a trauma survivor who falls within this category; I experience frequent, pervasive dissociation, and there are large portions of my life which I do not remember.

Perhaps the most well-known dissociative disorder is DID or dissociative identity disorder. DID is a condition which is often misunderstood and vilified, especially with portrayals in popular media. However, individuals with DID are no more dangerous than the average person and should be extended compassion and understanding just like all other trauma survivors. It involves having separate internal states – some people call these states *alters*, while others call them *parts*. They can be thought of as elements of one's personality, separated by the physical effects of trauma, and a person with DID may 'switch' (shift between parts/alters) according to the requirements of their day-to-day life.

What this looks like varies from person to person, and alters can form for a variety of reasons. Someone with DID may have an alter who is better at dealing with conflict, and so this may emerge during an argument. Another may appear for functional activities, such as getting dressed, or brushing one's teeth. It is important to note that this is not a delusion on the part of the person with DID: alters tend to be separated by dissociative and amnesic blocks.

It's not a perfect analogy but imagine if you had your six-year-old self, your fourteen-year-old self and your twenty-year-old self all in your head at once – and you couldn't control who is 'fronting' (making decisions and using the body). Although they are all you, they are distinct versions of you – with different likes, dislikes, ways of speaking and behaving, values and approaches to life. However, DID is rarely as dramatic as television makes it out to be. Although switches are involuntary, they are actually quite hard to notice, even if you know a person well: they can just look like mood swings or sudden bursts of confidence.

At its core, DID – much like all dissociative disorders – is a form of survival: a kind of ultra-compartmentalisation of one's thoughts, feelings and personality. Trauma survivors in general are very good at compartmentalising, and 'intellectualising' their thoughts rather than feeling their emotions. This is why DID and other trauma disorders can be very difficult to spot, even by trained professionals – we traumatised folk are often 'great' at therapy and know how to give all the right answers to protect ourselves. The first time a therapist noticed I was dissociating during a therapy session, I was overcome with an exceptional kind of anger: *Why did she have to point it out? I'm giving all the right answers; doesn't that mean I'm being good?*

Think of it this way: imagine you grew up in an environment where you needed to hold two conflicting opinions, simultaneously, to survive. For example: a child has a parent who is very frightening. This child may think, *My parent is supposed to take care of me. I love them.* This child may also think, *My parent hurts me. I'm angry at them and want to fight back.* It is thought that these ideas are too difficult to reconcile in a young brain, and so the brain does what it does best: it adapts. These two ideas become two modes for the traumatised person – two ways of behaving, two ways of thinking and feeling. It's almost like everyone is driving a car (the body), but when you dissociate to such an extreme level, there are several of you packed into the vehicle, taking turns at the wheel and all having different opinions on where and how to drive, or what music to play. An incredible, adaptive way of surviving – but exhausting and painful for the host if there is no support available.

Over time, these modes – which may begin simply as emotions or behaviours – can develop into their own parts or alters. Current research suggests that DID develops roughly between the ages of six and nine (around the time our personalities are solidifying), under specific traumatic pressure similar to that which results in CPTSD. Likewise, there is a blurry area between CPTSD and DID, which trauma researchers have unceremoniously dubbed 'OSDD', or other specified dissociative disorder: possessing issues with identity and chronic dissociative symptoms, but not quite fitting in one camp or the other. The truth is that trauma disorders are less a set of categories and more of a spectrum; experiences may differ greatly between two people with the same on-paper diagnosis.

I'm talking about this to give you a backdrop on the day-to-day life of a trauma survivor. There is no singular experience that can be quantified into one essay, but I feel this is a decent start to help understand why some of us may choose not to raise children. At the time of writing, my diagnosis is officially CPTSD with high dissociative tendencies.

The 'complex' in my CPTSD comes from the fact that my trauma began when I was very young, involved people I should have been able to trust, and was inescapable for a long time. No one survivor has a 'worse' condition than another: all treatments for trauma involve re-establishing that the world is a safe place to exist in. However, the reason that complex trauma warrants discussion, understanding and support is that we can't be told, 'The world isn't like this all of the time, so you don't need to be afraid anymore.' With complex trauma, our blueprint of the world isn't a default of kindness and joy. It's not even neutrality. It's just terror, and pain, and *survival*.

I have been in therapy for many years and will be for many more. Although I am no longer in the abusive, traumatic situations of my younger years, many of my days are spent in a whirl of sickness and pain. If you experienced trauma at seven years old and never had that terror resolved, when you're reminded of it, you're going to respond like you're the same age – with the emotional literacy of a child. It isn't that trauma survivors are incapable of logical thought, grounding or self-soothing; it's that often, our nervous systems are trapped in an anachronistic nightmare, ready to erupt at a moment's notice. We were robbed of our agency, independence and stability early on, and that loss haunts us throughout the rest of our lives.

Let's clear it up once and for all: having a trauma disorder does not make anyone an unfit parent. No one has ever been endangered by my trauma responses, and I am more than qualified to do the work I've done and continue to do. Indeed, I think my condition offers a unique perspective. I now support disabled and neurodivergent people in the arts and charity spaces, helping to write arts funding bids and working as a personal assistant. But having a child is another beast altogether. There is a huge difference between working with children in a controlled environment – where you can switch out who is taking responsibility and allow yourself a breather if you feel unwell – and being a child's primary caregiver. Having a trauma condition – or any mental health issue – does not mean someone will be abusive to their children, and such a notion is incredibly harmful to trauma survivors and our recovery.

On the other hand, recovery is a full-time job. It is not an intellectually stimulating thought experiment or an inspirational process to consume on social media. It's hard work, and it's *ugly*. Every parent who makes the decision to raise a child must take into account their own difficulties – whether they be financial constraints, physical issues, or a disability such as a trauma disorder.

We should not dissuade potential parents from having a child because they struggle with their health, whatever that looks like. What matters is that the parent can support the child. In my case, at my current stage of recovery, I know I couldn't. Everyone who has kids becomes overwhelmed from time to time, but there really aren't any days off from being a parent. I couldn't bundle off my child every time I have a flashback that leaves me zonked and puking . . . nor would I want to.

You can imagine why trauma survivors often feel selfish

prioritising our health and wellbeing. Many of us have trauma that required us to minimise our presence – to keep quiet, to perform duties as expected, and to push our way through abuse, neglect and terror with the stoic determination of a warrior. However, while raising a child absolutely requires a thankless kind of tenacity, such as forgoing sleep and leisure and all manner of joyful activities to ensure your child is safe and healthy, there is no honour in martyring yourself just to have the title of 'caregiver'. No one should try to raise a child just to fix their wounds.

Consider for a moment that your trauma – whatever it looks like – was a period of deprivation for you. Through no fault of your own, you experienced something no one should ever have to experience, and you don't need to spend your life apologising for the way that affects you. Even if you are biologically, financially or physically capable of raising a kid, *that does not mean you have to do so*. It's OK that I don't want to have kids. It's OK if you don't, either.

This is a rallying cry to all of my fellow trauma survivors, as well as to our allies, supporters, friends, family, loved ones – and those who just want to understand. If you do choose to have children, you are not a monster doomed to repeat the pain you have suffered in the past. You are a human being who deserves respect, empathy and understanding when you are in distress, and you can be an incredible parent.

Likewise, you are not abdicating responsibility if you choose not to have children; you are taking on the responsibility of healing your inner child. That is a journey that requires a tremendous amount of strength. You are not weak, and you're not a non-functioning adult. Whatever your situation and whatever your diagnosis, remember that every mood swing, panic attack and dissociative episode has its roots in protection. Recovery is not a straight line, and there will be days that are harder than others. But you have survived every single one of your bad days so far – and I know you can survive another.

Who knows? Maybe in ten years, I'll have changed my mind about having kids. For now, though, I'm just glad to see families in public and feel genuine happiness for them rather than experiencing a flashback. I know now that my worth is not dependent on how well I can take care of other people, children or otherwise. It isn't selfish to need time to heal. I hope, whatever your choice is, that you are able to take care of yourself first and foremost.

It does get easier.

I promise.

*Quinn Clark is an award-winning author, researcher and support worker. They live in Newcastle and are currently funded by Arts Council England, working on their debut full-length novel.*

# Decisions

*Sophia Money-Coutts*

It started when I was thirty-three, just after my boyfriend and I broke up. I'd blink at small children in the street, or babies strapped on women's chests in the park, and try to imagine having one. What would it feel like to be sitting on a bench, coffee in one hand, my other arm wrapped protectively around the papoose?

Some women seem to know instinctively that they want children. I never have. That's why I began testing myself as I approached my mid-thirties, as if squeezing an avocado in the supermarket for ripeness, squinting at other people's children while trying to gauge any reaction from my ovaries. Were they ripe? Did I want a baby? But no, nothing. No major response in either direction from my body. How unhelpful.

A year or so after that, I decided to freeze my eggs. I still didn't know whether I wanted a baby, but in the meantime I'd put my eggs on ice, while I was still relatively fertile, in case I wanted to use them down the line.

I've had more enjoyable experiences. Egg freezing, for me, meant a month of sniffing one chemical and injecting myself in the belly with another. It meant multiple trips to hospital and so many internal scans I lost count. It was the first summer of Covid, which meant hospitals were eerie and everyone was masked. It meant tears of frustration when I couldn't get the needle into my stomach, tears of loneliness at the idea that I was doing this to myself because I was single, then tears of fury when I felt selfish for complaining. Plenty of women couldn't afford to do this, I told myself, so get on with it.

I was lucky in the end, because my ovaries produced twenty-two eggs, which meant I didn't have to go through another round. That number, retrieved when I was thirty-five, gave me a 70 to 90 per cent chance of a baby in the future. No guarantee, but those seemed pretty good odds.

Phew, I thought, that's done. I can stop thinking about it.

Except I didn't stop thinking about it because it's very hard to ignore the question of children if you're a single woman in your mid-thirties. My friends were all having babies, Instagram showed me constant babies, alarmist *Daily Mail* headlines reminded me that the clock was ticking, and my mother talked increasingly often about her friends' grandchildren. Sometimes I wished my biological clock *had* kicked in. If I felt that desperate impulse, if I looked at a baby on the bus and my stomach went gooey, at least that would answer the question. But still . . . nothing. No yearning.

In the past few years, the term 'social infertility' has sprung up to describe women who long for children but haven't had them for social reasons, such as being single or unable to afford a baby, as opposed to medical reasons. I see this around me with certain single girlfriends; brilliant, vibrant, intelligent women who, for whatever reason, haven't found their person. But what I feel is less social infertility, and more indecision. Should I have a baby? Do I need to have a baby? Will I miss out if I don't have a baby? What if I don't have a baby and get to fifty and realise it's the biggest regret of my life? In America, they have therapists for women like me (course they do). Cough up a few hundred dollars in California and you can see a 'motherhood clarity mentor' to help answer these thorny questions.

The trouble was, after a couple of years getting over the break-up with the boyfriend mentioned above (I really wallow when it comes to break-ups), I was happy again. Finally, my heart was mended, stronger, and I loved being by myself again. I loved my South London flat; I loved waking up on a Saturday morning and being able to do exactly what I wanted to do. I could go to sleep when I wanted and fart in bed. Why would I wreck that by trying to find someone, by spending fruitless hours on dating apps, chasing a relationship simply because, if I *did* suddenly decide I wanted children, I had to find someone and – dreaded phrase – 'settle down'.

Not for me. So, last year, as I turned thirty-seven, I decided to try and forget about dating, to concentrate on work, on my writing, and travel after a couple of years of travel being so difficult. Selfish? Perhaps. But for most of my life, I've been a huge people pleaser, ignoring my own feelings or desires in order to make others happy, especially in relationships. Now I'd do what I wanted to do, not lose my sense of self in a relationship, or even think about children for a couple of years while I wrote and travelled and read books and went to crowded spaces like the theatre again and partied and generally celebrated after two years of life's currants being in short supply.

Obviously, then I met someone.

It was while spending a couple of months abroad and he was a wonderful if slightly chaotic man who ordered whisky after whisky on our first date and talked about American politics. After so long being determinedly single, I suddenly remembered how lovely it was to sit across from someone in a bar and feel recognition. I'd forgotten what it was like to stare longingly at my phone waiting for a message. I'd forgotten what it was like to think about my pants as a decorative item rather than purely functional. I'd forgotten what it was like to wake up and feel a chest against my back.

We saw one another a couple of times in London after that before he had to go abroad again for work.

A week or so later, I discovered I was pregnant.

I hesitate to call it an accident, as if it happened while I was crossing the road, because I don't want to sound flippant about pregnancy in a book discussing infertility. But it certainly wasn't planned. My initial reaction when I saw the test was to laugh in disbelief. Pregnant? But we only did it once that night, and I was thirty-seven, and I've had various gynaecological dramas in the past which made me assume getting pregnant would be difficult, and I wasn't very sure about him. And and and . . . I had a million ands.

Perhaps you played this game with friends in your twenties. If you got pregnant, what would you do? Back then, the answer was easy: become unpregnant as fast as possible. But at my age? The answer might have been trickier.

Except it wasn't. I knew immediately that I didn't want a baby. I still didn't know long-term whether I wanted them at all, but I definitely didn't want this one. I couldn't have a baby because I had books to write and not enough cash in the bank and I wasn't sure that a man who drank so much whisky and travelled so much father material.

What followed was a fraught three-week period of trying to sort the situation out. Referring to an abortion or termination as 'sorting the situation out' is coy, but the language is so charged and increasingly political that I found I could barely say the word 'abortion'. Two days after I found out I was pregnant, news broke in America that Roe v Wade might be overturned and I became obsessed with the story. I read every news article I could and listened to every podcast, trying to imagine what I'd feel like if I was sitting in Texas instead of the Early Pregnancy Unit at a South London hospital. Trapped and terrified, I surmised.

Every morning during this time, I'd wake and press a hand to my bare stomach, trying to feel any minute difference. It was a bit like the avocado test: did I feel any different today? Did I want this? I never did.

And it was confusing, early pregnancy. Or at least it was for me. My first two tests at home said I was pregnant, but one doctor sent me away and refused to help because his test was negative and he couldn't see anything on a scan. A week later, a different doctor confirmed that I was pregnant but he couldn't see anything on the scan, so perhaps I was miscarrying. Yet another week later, I was back at the hospital, where a nice nurse in blue scrubs confirmed that no no, I was pregnant, coming up for seven weeks, and pointed out the sac to me: a blob that looked like a small black grape clinging to my uterus.

I cried on the way home because I was so frustrated by this process, and hormonal, and because I *did* feel slightly guilty and ashamed for what I wanted to do to the little black grape. I hadn't instantly fallen in love with it, as tends to happen in films and books at such moments. Was there something wrong with me? Was I particularly cold, callous and unfeeling? Ironically, in my second novel, published three years earlier, my heroine Lil finds herself pregnant after a first date with a handsome adventurer who, by the time she takes the test, is halfway up a mountain in Asia. As soon as she has a six-week scan, she decides to keep it. But in my case, while the father of my baby was also abroad, I felt the opposite. Not now. Not like this.

In the end, a further week on, I found myself sitting outside a Marie Stopes clinic waiting room listening to sad panpipe music (note to MSI Reproductive Choices, which is what it's been rebranded as: you guys are doing the most heroic work but could we have different music at your clinics?). Half an hour later, a wonderfully kind and gentle nurse told me the little black grape was slipping away by itself and I cried yet again because I was so relieved. It wasn't straightforward and I had to return to the hospital three days later for an operation to clean me out. But at least it was resolved.

So, what's the lesson from all this? It's about choice, I reckon. I still don't know what I want long term. I have eggs on ice, which is a comfort, although they're no guarantee. I still want to write and travel. I still believe women are raised, subliminally, to think that the most important contribution we could make to the world is children, and that if we don't have them our lives will have been less meaningful. Motherhood remains a powerful form of identity (Mama jumpers, Mumsnet, cutesy Instagram pictures on Mother's Day), even if you're supposedly doing it badly (*Why Mummy Drinks*, the Scummy Mummies, *Motherland*), and if you're not part of that tribe, what even are you? That's why I remain so conscious of the question: should I have one? Do I really want one?

A while ago, a friend who's chosen not to have children emailed me after I wrote a piece about egg freezing. 'Don't have a baby!' she wrote. 'It's like smokers wanting people not to give up on the theory there's only so much lung cancer to go round, so the more smokers, the more the risk is diluted. I want everyone to stop having kids so that I don't want to have one!'

I admire this friend, and am a tiny bit jealous of her, for knowing so clearly what she wants when I still don't. But slowly I'm relaxing into my ambivalence, and wonder whether I've considered this more than some people who plunge into parenthood? Perhaps my future has my own children in it; perhaps it doesn't. Perhaps I'll go one way and love a small person more ferociously than I would have thought possible; perhaps I'll simply love my nieces and nephews. Perhaps I won't even be able to get pregnant again. That, too, is something I think about. Who knows? But I'm grateful that we (in the UK) have more choice than our own mothers. If choosing to have children is OK, then so is not choosing to. None of this is easy, but I'm grateful that, thus far at least, the decisions have been mine.

*Sophia Money-Coutts is an award-winning journalist and newspaper columnist, and the author of five novels.*

# 'Happy Ending'

### *Seetal Savla*

I am on the verge of becoming a 'success story' and I don't know how to feel about it. Within the next fortnight, I hope to bring home our baby. After our gruelling six-year fertility journey, this will be a 'happy ending'. Neither label sits well with me. When they crop up in conversation, I have to resist an overwhelming urge to remind the well-meaning relative/friend/acquaintance of what my husband and I have endured to get to this point. Focusing solely on the joy of this unexpected pregnancy is to gloss over the turmoil – emotional, mental, physical and financial – of our previous attempts to conceive.

Over the course of trying to conceive, I had gone through natural pregnancy resulting in an early miscarriage; four failed fresh IVF cycles using our own eggs and sperm at three London-based fertility clinics (one NHS and two private); a cancelled donor-egg IVF cycle and then successful donor-egg IVF with a different donor followed by a brutal missed miscarriage in the first trimester. Then, suddenly, I was pregnant. No medications, transvaginal scans, regular monitoring or procedures were required this time – nature had somehow achieved this seemingly unobtainable feat all on her own.

I have heard countless 'success stories' over the years, particularly when I've announced yet another failed cycle. At my most vulnerable, in desperate need of expressing my anger and hopelessness, I would be greeted by a wall of toxic positivity. My messy words and feelings were not welcome; they made people feel awkward and inadequate, and who wants to feel that way? What these storytellers wanted to hear was that I would 'keep going!', just like their cousin/colleague/ etc. did, until I too was rewarded for my efforts. If I ended my journey without a baby, I knew they would see me as weak; someone who gave up too easily and too soon, who 'did not want it enough'. A failure to be treated with pity in our pronatalist society, which favours pregnancy and birth above all.

These stories did not inspire but trigger me – they still do. I found them infuriating because the longer we tried, the further we got from success and that made me loathe myself. Not only was my body repeatedly refusing to do what nature had intended, it was failing to respond to the best medical interventions. For some, having faith in a higher power can offer comfort during the depths of their despair. It can also make it easier to accept the cruel cards that some of us are dealt because they are 'part of God's plan'.

Growing up, Hinduism was a huge part of my life, but my relationship with religion has changed during adulthood for several reasons, the main one being my husband's atheism. Although I would still describe myself as Hindu, I am no longer a practising one; at least, not in the sense of daily prayers, a home shrine, regular temple visits and marking the major events in our lunar calendar through lengthy religious ceremonies.

My much-needed hope came in the form of the 'childless not by choice' community on Instagram. I can see you wondering how people without children can inspire someone yearning to build a family, but I wanted to know that I would be OK if we called time on Project Baby. I needed to see real-life examples and find new role models. I started to explore what it might feel like to prioritise the life we had now over a life we might have. I was under no illusions and knew that the road to acceptance would be difficult in a different way from becoming a parent, a slow transition rather than an immediate switch, but I loved seeing how the community's amazing advocates succeeded in redefining joy in their lives. Hearing these stories was reassuring to me in a way that pregnancy stories were not.

Six years separated my first pregnancy from my third and current one, and my reactions could not have been more different. On Christmas Day 2015, I shouted with delight when 'pregnant' appeared on the digital test. Clutching that life-changing piece of plastic, I rushed into the bedroom to share the news with my stunned husband. I climbed into bed, pulled the duvet over our heads, and enthusiastically projected our future. Just like that, all the fears that I had expected to feel in this moment evaporated – losing my identity, independence and figure – but also my uncertainty about whether I actually wanted to be a mother or whether I was feeling the pressure to procreate from certain family members and our South Asian community.

My husband took a more pragmatic approach. Conscious of what could go wrong, he preferred to wait and see how the pregnancy progressed before allowing himself to fully embrace it. Not once did miscarriage cross my mind. How I envy that naive version of myself now. That brief, precious pregnancy gave me a glimpse of something I thought I did not want, made me realise how much I did desire it, and promptly ripped it away from me. Our first loss stripped me of my innocence. I knew that if I ever became pregnant again, there would be no unbridled elation.

So eight months ago, on a nondescript Monday evening, when the second blue line on the pregnancy test became visible, I felt numb. I had not even wanted to buy the test because for the first time ever on this journey, living in uncertainty felt safer than knowing the truth. There was no excited expletive this time, just a quiet grunt as if to say: 'Here we go again. How far will we get this time?'

Having the pregnancy confirmed by my gynaecologist and seeing the gestational sac on screen did not make me any happier. The image seemed as though it belonged to someone else – maybe a training video had accidentally been left on? Hope had made such a fool of me before that I could not allow myself to believe this embryo, made from one of my own 'poor quality' forty-year-old eggs, would be the one to make it.

I found it impossible to connect with the miracle that was happening inside my body. Although I yearned to savour every moment and every symptom, I had to protect myself. At least, that is what I told myself, all while knowing that it was an exercise in futility. No amount of preparing for the worst in theory can prepare you for the reality.

We had swapped London for Berlin in late 2020 (because Brexit) and, when we visited family and friends during my first trimester, a considerable advantage of our unsuccessful fertility track record was that no one suspected a thing. There were no sly glances when I politely declined alcoholic drinks, no jumping to conclusions. I enjoyed having this secret and, for the first time in several years, I felt some semblance of control.

In an ideal world, I would have guarded my precious secret until the very end and stayed in Berlin to work through my anxieties with my therapist. This might seem extreme, but I had to brace myself to deal with how people would react to our surprise pregnancy. We would be heartily congratulated, told to stay positive, and encouraged to enjoy this long-awaited experience. There's nothing wrong with any of these reactions as such, but when the focus is entirely on the happy ending, it becomes even more important for my past trauma and losses to be acknowledged and for our angel babies' short lives to be honoured.

South Asian communities excel at sweeping awkward subjects under the carpet, especially those related to women's bodies, due to the shame and stigma still associated with them. I knew that our news would instantly erase all the failures and miscarriages from people's minds. Conversations from this point onwards would be upbeat, staying well within everyone's comfort zones. Why keep harping on about the ugliness of the past when you have almost achieved your goal? Because we know how quickly our fragile hearts can be broken and our delicate dreams obliterated.

We finally shared our secret around the twenty-week mark, when it was becoming increasingly difficult to explain why we would not be attending birthdays and weddings. I was also feeling immensely disingenuous about carrying on private conversations with people about their fertility battles without disclosing my significant news. The longer I left it, the stronger the likelihood became of it doing irreparable damage to these friendships by breaching trust.

While it would have been simpler to post a single announcement on all my social media feeds to inform everyone, I did not entertain that idea for long. The thought of one of my friends seeing such news and being triggered was intolerable. Having been sent compassionate private messages by others prior to them going public, I was keen to pay this kind act forward.

Being on this side of the fence made me understand how challenging it must have been for people to tell me they were having a baby, especially when they had not been trying to conceive. I did not want to cause anyone pain, but I was cognisant that it was inevitable, with the surprise natural pregnancy element being the real kicker.

My therapist and I often explored this 'survivor's guilt' during our sessions. She helped me to see that even though this feeling was completely normal in the circumstances, I was not responsible for others' reactions. Carrying their struggles in addition to my own was self-defeating. All I could do was be considerate, give them the space to digest this unexpected development, and understand that they may not be able to interact with me, online or offline, for some time. Just as I had made use of the mute and unfollow functions on social media to protect myself from bump, birth and baby photos, I knew many would tap those buttons to avoid mine.

As with any major life changes, my pregnancy has impacted my friendships to varying degrees. These are tricky waters to navigate: we may want to continue to support one another, but when there is suffering and endless setbacks on one side and guilt and muted joy on the other, the best short-term solution is often to maintain distance. I only hope that a bit of breathing space does not lead to a permanent separation.

Interestingly, some other friendships have also been affected. In the aftermath of my miscarriage, once my daily desire to stare at a screen and drown my sorrows had passed, I needed people to rage at the unfairness and cruelty of the world with me. Instead, some could only operate in practical mode, telling me that I could try again, that I should be strong, that time would heal me. Those basic, frustrating platitudes were akin to a door being shut and locked, leaving me in dark solitude. The door still allowed small talk to filter through the cracks, but who wants to talk about the weather and the week ahead when their baby has just died? I certainly did not. A year later, I still have these unrewarding inconsequential conversations with them because the door remains locked and none of us can remember where we kept the key.

I know how fortunate I am to have supportive family and friends, but I know now that not everyone has the capacity to offer the empathy and compassion I need. Expecting them to change is unrealistic and only hurts me. I will always be grateful for those who held, and still hold, space for me to express my feelings without judgement or trying to fix me. Without them, the occasional moments of isolation that I still feel would be more frequent. The most comforting comments wished us 'gentle/cautious/quiet congratulations' and validated our complex feelings.

It is also possible to receive too much support, especially

when you do not find that support to be particularly comforting. The check-ins and calls can feel suffocating, which leads to guilt because you should be feeling grateful for this kindness. It is often at its strongest in the first few months after a loss, when the person who is grieving wants to know that people care, that their loss matters to others, but also wants to be left alone to process their pain without the predictable toxic positivity.

I confided in friends in a similar position who gently encouraged me to lean into moments of joy as and when they come. Many told me that they wished they had been able to enjoy their pregnancies more, which made me realise that, if this was to be my only full-term pregnancy, I wanted to cherish it. I wanted to stay grounded in the present and focus on what was real instead of catastrophising.

After months of pulling ourselves back from thinking too far ahead to minimise our anxieties, we find ourselves reflecting on the next steps for our family. In parallel to prioritising Baby Savla's safe arrival into the world, we have been tentatively dipping our toes back into the donor-conception waters by deciding how to proceed regarding the two embryos patiently waiting for us in a freezer at our London clinic.

Could we put ourselves through another frozen-embryo transfer for a shot at giving our child a sibling? As I would be in my early forties at this point and our chances of success would be diminishing by the day, how would we cope with a potential failure? On the bright side, if we were successful, how would our biological child and donor-conceived child relate to one another, and to us? But if treatment is off the table, what would happen to these embryos?

Our surprise natural pregnancy has allowed us to avoid

answering these questions for a little longer, but we cannot do so indefinitely. If we choose not to pursue any further treatment, there are two main options: discard the embryos or donate them. Having financially and emotionally invested in these cherished cells, saying goodbye to them at this stage would feel like a tremendous waste to us. Similarly, undergoing a compassionate transfer – transferring the embryos when pregnancy is less likely to occur – would be unsuitable in our case.

Which leads us onto donation to another woman or couple, or to medical research. The former takes us into complicated territory. On the one hand, we would be giving someone struggling to conceive the opportunity to build their much-wanted family (provided that our egg donor has consented and we meet the eligibility criteria in the UK). In view of our challenges, it would be a privilege to give this beautiful gift to someone. However, if we decided against more treatment and then someone became pregnant using our embryo, how would that sit with us? It is much easier to part with something precious when the implications of your generosity have yet to materialise. We can hypothesise about how this pregnancy and subsequent baby would impact us, but the truth is that we can never truly know until it becomes reality.

A successful outcome would also mean that my husband would have a biological baby in whose life he would not be involved, at least not unless the child wishes to contact him when they reach eighteen – anonymous donations were possible in the UK until 2005, when the law changed to allow donor-conceived people to have access to their donor's name, date of birth and last known address. Even if we opted out of learning whether a baby was conceived via our donation, we would wonder what happened and whether they would want to initiate contact one day. We would also need to consider when and how we would share this part of our story with our child. Hiding the truth from them would not be an option. We chose a non-anonymous donor so that our potential donor-conceived child could fully trace their biological roots and would therefore be transparent with our biological child about the possibility of them having half-siblings.

Donating our embryos to science would enable us to side-step this emotional minefield. Researchers would use them to increase their knowledge and develop treatments for serious diseases, look into new fertility treatments, learn more about the causes of miscarriages and more. Knowing that we had made a valuable contribution to medical research in this field would give us a great sense of satisfaction and be a worthwhile way to close this chapter of our lives.

For the time being, though, we have the luxury of postponing this decision, at least for six months or so. Over the next fortnight, our immediate focus is the safe arrival of our sweet surprise and finding our feet as first-time parents to a living baby. While our initial fears and anxieties centred around suffering another loss, these have recently been replaced with ones concerning the birth. I had assumed that after years of living in limbo, I would be adept at navigating these new unknowns; instead, I find myself fretting about them. As with the decision about our remaining embryos, it is almost impossible to predict how we will react to certain situations when they do eventually arise. Whatever happens, both with the baby in my belly and the shape of our future family, this is not an ending but the beginning of a new chapter in our story.

In any case, none of us knows what the future holds. Our fertility journey has taught us to take life one step at a time because what we know right now is all we know for sure. Sharing my story also showed me that I'm not alone or abnormal, feelings that can easily consume you when you keep your struggles to yourself. The kind messages I have received over the years from those who have invested in our journey have pulled me through some of my darkest days. There is such power in solidarity. These conversations encouraged me to be more compassionate towards myself over time and allowed me to accept that however our attempts to have a baby panned out, I would survive, and eventually thrive.

My plan now is to apply these valuable lessons and experiences to the imminent birth of our baby and subsequent steps into parenthood. If and when the situations we worry about present themselves, we will figure it out. Such is life.

*Seetal Savla is a freelance writer and fertility advocate working to break the stigma surrounding infertility, especially within South Asian communities. She has an MA in Audiovisual Translation Studies, and after living in Paris and Montreal for several years, she is now based in Berlin with her husband Neil and their rainbow baby, Meghna. You can continue to follow her journey on Instagram @SavlaFaire.*

# Parenting

# Self-Portrait, Pregnant

## Miranda Ward

I

*2022*

There's a painting of a pregnant woman that I keep returning to: a self-portrait by the artist Ghislaine Howard, made in 1984, shortly before the birth of her first child. In the painting, a woman sits, her head resting against one hand, the other in her lap, drawing the viewer's attention to the bulge of her belly. The colours are simple: muted yellows, whites, the blue of a coat or dressing gown. The subject's face is indistinct, but there's a weariness in her posture, a kind of contemplative exhaustion – in an article published in *The Artist* magazine in 1986, Howard draws a comparison between her portrait and Dürer's *Melencolia I*, a similarity which she herself only noticed in retrospect.

What I'm attracted to in this image, what keeps me coming back again and again is the mundanity of it, the plainness of it. The pregnant woman in this painting is not a hero, not a villain, not a paragon of beauty or placid maternity or strength and virtue. She is, in fact, and appropriately, unfinished:

'Just when I felt my work was going well,' Howard writes, 'life rudely interrupted art when my son Maxim was born almost a month earlier than expected and the large oil painting that I had only just begun remained unfinished. And so it is today.'

The other thing I'm attracted to in this image is its very existence, the simple fact of it having been made. In this respect it represents an act of courage. To me personally, I mean. The courage of a pregnant woman to document her pregnancy, to make something of it even before its outcome can be known. To proclaim it, stake a claim in it, own and accept it.

## II
*20 weeks*
*February 2020*

In the waiting room for the anatomy scan, I sit on a hard plastic chair and fill out a form.

*How many pregnancies, including this one, have you had?* the form asks.

I hesitate; it feels strange to write it down, it seems false, as if I might be accused of lying. *But they weren't* real *pregnancies,* a voice in my head tells me, a voice that sounds suspiciously like my own. *They don't count.* Except that medically they do. Medically speaking, it is necessary, at this juncture, to write them down.

5, I write, using the cheap biro the receptionist gave me when I said I didn't have a pen on me. Five. It looks wrong, it looks like too many. Have I miscalculated? I count on my fingers: *miscarriage, miscarriage, ectopic, miscarriage,* and now – *this.* Five. A full hand.

*How many children do you have?* the form asks.

*0,* I write.

*So far,* I add, in my head. I've been trying to let go of the superstitions, of the rituals of control I know, logically, have no bearing on what happens in this pregnancy, but it's harder than it sounds. Sometimes, still, I have to allow myself to believe that I have the power to write my own future, if only I want it enough, if only I can curtail my impulses. I have to look away from the maternity clothes in the shop, the baby clothes, *not yet, not yet,* play little games of denial and deceit, *just in case.*

After I finish filling out the form I wait to be called in for the scan. They're running a few minutes behind schedule. While I sit, my back straight, my legs crossed, my small bump obscured under a large jumper, I think of the number *five.* Of the ghost timelines. All the other ways it could have been.

Throughout this pregnancy I've felt I've been haunting myself. Each time I reach another private milestone – a point at which I've miscarried previously, a missed due date, appointments and scans I've had before, or had to cancel – I feel simultaneously bound to my past and liberated from it, as if I'm two people, or three or four or an infinite number of people, all at once. Each time I find myself in a familiar place, a room where I've sat before, a consultant's office or hospital car park, I'm keenly aware of the ghost of myself. I've found it hard to take up space during this pregnancy, to assert myself as *pregnant,* but also to assert myself at all, and perhaps it's because I feel I'm already taking up so much space. Here I am in the waiting room on this chair, but also on that one and that one, and that one. Here I am, here I am, here I am already, everywhere I go, not an I at all but a *we*.

## III
*5 weeks*
*October 2014*

*Here we are.* Two lines on a plastic stick. That's how it starts, that's how it always starts, no matter how it ends.

At the beginning a pregnancy is just an idea. It's a thing that isn't quite, a thing you can't see or touch or hear, a thing you have to put your faith in without any real proof of its existence.

Well, isn't that what faith is?

I suppose there is proof, of a sort. The two lines on the plastic stick. The whisper of nausea as you wash your hands, the smell of the soap too strong, too cloying. (I'll never again be able to use Pears without thinking of this moment, without feeling, briefly, definitely *pregnant*.)

After the test I lie down on my bed, though it's only mid-afternoon. I have more work to do; I have onions and chopped tomatoes to pick up from the shop, an evening to fill. I'm not tired, or am I? I feel the same as I did this morning, but different, too. I'd planned to go for a run later but already it feels as if I'm slipping away from that person; I'm someone else now; my muscles feel softer, more pliable, my body buzzing and compliant, attuned to its own rhythms.

*Here we are, here we are, here we are.*

*Here* is only a moment in time, of course. Every place, every body, is just a snapshot of itself. Every place, every body, is also an archive of itself. It holds its own history. It holds its own futures, too, all of them – the ones that will come to pass, and the ones that won't. Every place, every body, is a possibility waiting to happen. The space between those lines is an invitation I don't know how to accept, because to do so means, also, to accept – not only to acknow-ledge but *accept* – whatever might come next. *Whatever might come next.*

## IV
*7 weeks*
*March 2016*

I've never seen a heartbeat before. It's not even a heartbeat; the embryo's heart isn't yet fully formed, it's just a flutter where the heart will be, but that's how the nurse phrases it – *a heartbeat* – and so that's how I start to think of it, too.

I've been bleeding. Just like last time. As I pull down my tights, my underwear, slide onto the bed with my bum on the edge in preparation for the internal ultrasound, I tell the nurse I'm pretty sure I know what to expect, that it won't be good news. I try to soften the blow not for my own sake (I tell myself) but for hers, so that she won't have to scramble for the right words, won't have to feel as if she's dousing the flame of my hope – but then there it is, flashing on the screen, the heartbeat, the flutter, *a good sign*, she says, smiling reas-suringly. She seems excited to share this with us, to give us good news. I suppose a lot of her job is giving people good news, but a lot of it is also giving people news they don't want to hear. I suppose that later, when she finishes her shift, when she gets home and kicks her Crocs off and sits on the sofa cradling a cup of tea and switches on the television, she'll be thinking of the people to whom she had to deliver the bad news. Me she won't remember, not really. I'm a light moment in her day, a relief: a strange role to cast myself in. Not the one I expected, *given my history*, I'd said, by which I only meant *given the thing that happened last time, which might or might not happen again.*

In the waiting room, before the scan, before I knew the embryo was still growing – for now – I'd had my first real flash of insight into how many different versions of this story there could be. There I sat, a happily pregnant woman; there I sat, a woman miscarrying; there I sat, both at once. *A double life*, I'd thought.

## V

*12 weeks*
*March 2019*

Twelve is the magic number, isn't it? At twelve weeks you're supposed to be able to breathe out a sigh of relief and upload your scan photo to Instagram with a cute caption.

*We've been working on a little something . . .*
*Coming this summer!*
*Some, as they say, \*personal\* news . . .*

(Let me tell you something that perhaps doesn't paint me in a very sympathetic light: even though this story, my story, has a baby at the end of it, even though it should no longer matter to me, still I feel an instinctive, residual squeeze of panic, of rage and envy and self-loathing, whenever I see one of those photos. Even now, even years later, even if it's just for a second, I think: *how dare you.*)

Three days ago, at twelve weeks exactly, we saw one of those images for the first time – a grainy transformation of echoes that looked recognisably like a *baby*, or at least like the promise of one. Feet, hands, a button nose. I'd been bleeding again but everything was fine – *look, the heartbeat, look, a lovely clear image, we'll print it out for you*, and they did. I tucked it in my notebook and stopped at the Co-op on the way home to buy extra-thick pads to soak up the blood.

But now here I am again, in a familiar place: the bleeding hasn't stopped; the bleeding, in fact, has got worse; I've bled through the extra-thick pads and stained the passenger seat of our car and I have this photograph tucked in my notebook that proves something and nothing all at once. *Here we are. Here we are again.*

As I sit, waiting for my dating scan, I feel like a fraud. I shouldn't be here, I think. I'm not like the other women, stroking their bellies, planning for the future, even though there's a version of this story where I am, or could be.

(And how am I to know, in this moment, that almost exactly a year later I'll be here again, in this very room, waiting for an anatomy scan, filling in a form, counting my pregnancies on one hand?)

A nurse calls me in; *lie back*, the cold gel, the decisive movement of the wand, *I'm sorry*, she says, but I don't need her to tell me, I can see it, stark as anything: the lighthouse heartbeat that had been there three days ago blinking at me, a beacon of hope, isn't there now. I can see it, even before I feel it, before I know it.

## VI
*16 weeks*
*January 2020*

I think about this a lot, these days: the (in)visibility of pregnancy; what isn't shown, what can't be shown. *She's showing,* you might say of a woman you know to be pregnant, by which you might mean that beneath her clothes now a certain shape is discernible. But showing what, exactly? And if something is being shown, what else is being hidden; what is being obscured?

Was I really pregnant, all those times before, I wonder? What do I have to *show* for it?

I'm showing now, but I'm not. It's January and I'm wearing long jumpers and loose dresses that give nothing away, though I have to leave my jeans unbuttoned, and my T-shirts are getting tight. I'm teaching a course at the local university and sometimes I wonder if my students can tell, if they can see it yet. If they can see it when I stand in front of them in the lecture theatre, and all their eyes are trained on me, and I am trying to project a certain image of myself that doesn't necessarily match the way I feel – an image of myself as confident, knowledgeable, undaunted by their youth, their unfettered curiosity, which sometimes pulls me up short; *I don't know,* I find myself saying in answer to their questions, too often. *I don't know, I don't know. What a great question.*

At first I thought, a little defensively, *so what if they can see that I'm pregnant?* But then, also, I thought: *I* want *them to see that I'm pregnant.*

And why? Why should it matter if they do or do not witness my pregnancy, notice it, consider it?

*I don't know. What a great question.*

## VII
*6 weeks*
*August 2016*

Sometimes what you can't see might kill you. I had understood this, abstractly, about illness, about the ways in which the invisible processes of our bodies can become dangerous without our knowing, but I had not thought about it in terms of pregnancy before. I had thought, for a long time, of pregnancy as a binary state: you were either pregnant or not; it was simple, it was black and white, even though my experience was anything but simple. But now I am sort of pregnant, I am pregnant but not really, I am pregnant according to the test – two lines on a plastic stick – but the levels of hCG in my blood are not rising at the right rate; in fact, they're not rising at all. An ectopic pregnancy is suspected, but can't be confirmed yet. The embryo is always unviable with an ectopic pregnancy, and if left untreated it can cause rupture, internal bleeding, death. In other words, I may or may not be walking around with a ticking time bomb in my body. It may or may not go off at any moment. This is pregnancy too, you know, though it's hard to hold that in your mind when the only version of pregnancy you've ever really seen represented is characterised by a warm glow, a gentle swelling, the comic waddle and heavy, happy sighs of anticipation so beloved by filmmakers.

After work, to still my mind, I stroll up the hill to a park near our house. It's summer, warm, a wind moving the branches of the trees as I look out towards the city skyline, the cranes and spires. Even caught in a web of unknowing, it's possible to perceive the beauty of the evening, though whether this brings comfort or not I can't say. When, a week later, a scan shows what we've all suspected, an empty womb, a pregnancy out of place, when I'm scheduled for emergency surgery, when I emerge from the haze of anaesthesia minus one fallopian tube, my body tender and my brain wired, I feel, among other things, a sense of relief. To know for certain. To not have, for once, to think of anything other than myself, my recovery. To understand a little better the shades of nuance around not just pregnancy itself but also my own desire, where it begins and ends.

## VIII
*24 weeks*
*March 2020*

I'll tell you something else that perhaps doesn't paint me in a very sympathetic light. For all the years that I struggled to get pregnant, or stay pregnant, a small red part of me craved most of all not a baby but simply the *visibility* of a pregnant body, the attention it garners, the respect, envy, admiration, the sheer space it can take up. Tired of folding myself up on the Tube or in crowds, always making myself smaller and smaller, I wanted to be so large, so solid, that others would have to move around *me* for a change. Would notice me, notice, with respect, my swollen belly, my pumped-up breasts. I think often of the scene in *The Argonauts* where Maggie Nelson describes being saluted by members of the armed services as she moves, pregnant, through an airport, even though the point of that scene is also to call attention to the ways in which society fears and reviles a pregnant body. In my selfishness, in my obsessive desire to hold on to a pregnancy, I have often forgotten that part of the story, have fixated instead on the aspiration: to be saluted; no, simpler than that, to be *seen*, acknowledged, witnessed in my pregnant state.

I am trying now to understand how to ascribe public significance to those pregnancies which I have carried, however briefly, that went unseen, unnoticed, unsaluted. *Was I really pregnant all those times before?*

We're in Paris, my husband and I, sleeping on the couch in an Airbnb our friend has rented in the Marais, crashing her holiday because, we think giddily, we won't be able to do this so easily when the baby comes (*if*, says the small voice in my head that I can't quite silence). The couch is bright orange and sports a series of ambiguous stains that I try not to think about each night. I sleep lightly, and only on my left side now, with a pillow tucked between my legs, my hips and lower back aching by the morning.

This evening we're near the Sorbonne, at a restaurant, eating pasta. I take a few sips of red wine, warm and smooth on my tongue. Earlier this morning we walked past Notre-Dame, the shell of it, ringed by boards explaining the damage and how, in time, it would be repaired and rebuilt. I remembered the night it burned, a few weeks after miscarrying again, the way I watched the video clips on Twitter and felt utterly undone by the sight of it, even though I had no personal connection to the place, no reason in particular to mourn its loss.

At the restaurant, I excuse myself to go to the toilet. It's early March, still cold outside, but inside it's warm and I've shrugged off my coat. Underneath is a tight black maternity dress that I allowed myself to purchase ahead of this trip, a dress I know makes me look visibly, noticeably pregnant, no mistake about it.

True: since we've arrived I've spent a tense half hour on the phone to my midwife, seeking reassurance that in the end she cannot give me, because no one can ever guarantee that everything is going to be alright. True: every time I go to the toilet, still, I look first for any sign of blood. True: I've tried and failed to perceive a rhythm to the baby's kicks, even though I know it's too early to do so. I've anxiously consulted the NHS list of foods to avoid during pregnancy so often that I know it by heart and still find myself fretting over the details. (*Is Comté unpasteurised? Does it matter?*) But as I descend the stairs towards the bathroom and a waiter passes, heading up, I allow myself a moment of peace, a moment of being a pregnant body in public, of imagining that the waiter has noticed, and – the greatest luxury of all, perhaps – thought nothing of it. Thought, perhaps, *just another pregnant woman with a weak bladder.*

Later we'll go to a bar nearby; the floors will be sticky and my lemonade will taste vaguely of chlorine; in one corner a jazz flautist will strike up. In spite of all this, or perhaps because of it, the sticky floors, the chlorine taste, the jazz flute, the stains on the bright orange couch, even in spite of the tense call with my midwife, the instinctive clutch of fear that grabs me occasionally, I'll feel for a moment as if I'm floating, as if perhaps it is possible, after all, to repair and rebuild.

## IX
*5 weeks*
*October 2019*

*Here we are. Here we are. Here we are.*

Two lines, an invitation. At what point do you allow your-self the luxury of hope, the luxury of imagining a particular future?

I say luxury, but perhaps it's not. Perhaps it's a necessity, the *necessity* of hope.

An October afternoon, damp and chill. I finish my lecture and head for the toilets. There it is: a smear of blood, a famil-iar wave of disappointment, of resignation. I stare at the scuffed toes of my silver brogues, notice a ladder in my tights.

*Maybe this time will be different.*

*Maybe it won't.*

*Maybe it will.*

What I didn't know, what I've never known when I saw those lines, was this: whether, at the end of this pregnancy, I would have a baby or not, a *live birth*, as the fertility clinic phrases it. You can never know that about a pregnancy; there is no way to know, there is no way to account for all possible outcomes.

Possibility seems such a full word, but I've learned it can be an empty one, too. A possibility can be anything, and so, by implication, also nothing. It's a whisper, a ghost, a hope; it's full of air. When you've lived for so long, as I have done, in what I've come to think of as *the meantime country*, want-ing and waiting and trying and trying and trying, possibility can be a prison, or a poison. It can cause you to languish for too long in that mean place, to spend tens of thousands of pounds you may or may not have on treatments that may or may not work; it can taint your relationship with your body, with your family, your friends, your partner. For all that it has no substance, possibility can be a weight, an endless wait.

And yet: here we are. Still, again. Here we are. If I'm wondering, now, where the proof of those other pregnancies is, how I honour those other ways it could have been while also being intensely grateful for the way it is or might still be, then perhaps I need look no further, perhaps this is it: the capacity for gratitude, the capacity for hope, the conviction, as I walk down the hill in an autumn mist, that one way or another it will be alright.

# X
## 2022

All through my pregnancy with my son I resisted documenting it, visually or otherwise. I resisted naming him. I did not write about it, except abstractly, in code, allusion, never directly. I did not take selfies in the mirror as my body changed. Towards the end of the pregnancy it occurred to me that I might like a photograph of my bump unclothed, a photograph just for me, proof of something, but I never took it. I kept thinking, *I'll wait a bit longer* – that grasp at control, always, the denials, the deals. When, at thirty-five weeks and three days pregnant, I was admitted to the hospital after my waters broke, I thought, *I should take that photo now*, but still I didn't. I thought it the afternoon I went into labour, before I really understood what was happening; but *no*, I thought, *I'll do it tomorrow perhaps – not yet, not yet*. And then by tomorrow the baby – like Howard's, a month earlier than expected – had come, and I had missed my moment, had moved on to other things, to the business, the sleeplessness, of mothering a newborn.

*Was I really pregnant?* Sometimes, even after everything, even after the birth itself, I still wondered it; still felt unseen, unsaluted, unacknowledged, and so in some small way untruthful. But the answer to that question is, unlike most things about pregnancy, simple. *Yes*. With or without documentation, with or without a live birth, a heartbeat, a scan photo to post on Instagram, with or without witnesses and soldiers saluting, I was pregnant; I have been pregnant. Five times, *so far*.

So, here we are, and here is what I know – here, in the end, is all I know – on this subject: pregnancy is a plural thing. When I say *we* in this essay I mean, yes, me and the baby who could have been, the baby who might be. I mean me and the embryo that became my son, who lodged himself, breech, in my ribcage, so that by the end I could find no way to be comfortable; who arrived early in the midst of the hot, eerie May of 2020, a tiny creature with dark hair and an indignant shout; who grew and grew, too big for the clothes we brought him home in, too big for the clothes we'd just bought him; who learned to roll over and crawl and walk and talk and say to me one morning, *Let's talk about dreams*; who I'm late, right now, to pick up from nursery. But also: me and myself. Me and all the ghost timelines, me and all the ways it has been, it hasn't been, it might have been, it is, it could be or might be or will be or won't be. Me and all the versions of myself, in all these different stories.

*Miranda Ward is a freelance writer, editor and lecturer. She has a PhD in Cultural Geography from Royal Holloway, University of London, and is particularly interested in the relationship between space, place and the body. She grew up on a cattle ranch in California and now lives in Oxford. Her memoir* Adrift: Fieldnotes from Almost-Motherhood, *was published in 2021.*

# The Baby-Loss Diaries

*Nana-Adwoa Mbeutcha*

## Friday, 14 September 2018

The kids are in bed. I don't know what to say to Donald. I don't even know what to think. You know my baby. The baby is dead. Today has been such a weird day. Dead. How?

So, you know that hernia I have. Can't remember the proper name. The one I got during my labour with Gabriel I think, where my tummy muscles separated, or something like that. Well today it was hurting soooo badly. I could barely walk or talk. Donald was at work and Mum went home last night. I called her this morning to come back and look after the kids so I could go to A&E, but strangely, she just kept saying, 'Call your husband to come home, he needs to be there.' Although it was said in a loving way, I found it odd coz normally she would just drop everything and come. So anyway, I didn't argue coz yes, I should have called my 'husband' first. Donald left work and came straight home. By the time he got here I was feeling much better, and I actually had a routine midwife appointment in the afternoon so I thought, 'Perfect. I can go to the appointment without the kids, coz they're now four, three and eighteen months, so going with them was going to be hassle anyway.' But, Donald being Donald, and loving to do things as a family any time the opportunity arises, insisted he and the kids come with me. And thank God they did.

Today was going to be the first time I heard my baby's heartbeat. It was my eighteen-week appointment and I think it's quite normal to wait until then. I can't actually remember what happened with the others. I remember lying on the bed as the midwife put that cold jelly stuff on my tummy and started to rummage that heartbeat detector thing over it.

I don't really feel like writing anymore. Goodnight.

### Saturday, 15 September 2018

I've been walking around with a dead baby inside me. Yesterday the midwives kept asking me, 'Had you started feeling movement?' I thought I had . . . little flutterings here and there. I'm so sure I did on Thursday night. I remember sitting on the sofa and feeling that little sense of peace and excitement that I was finally feeling my baby moving. Maybe the baby was dead but still floating around. I dunno. The doctor said that it seems, from the scan, that the baby had only just died, as the placenta looks so fresh. But another doctor said my baby died two weeks earlier, which they could tell because of her or his size. So yeah, baby is dead and I can't quite believe this is happening. For as long as I can remember I have always been one to imagine awful things, but I can't believe this has actually happened. I spent a lot of time in bed and left Donald to look after the other three. I don't really know how he's feeling.

Maybe they've made a mistake. Doctors aren't always right.

Monique asked me if she could pray that the baby would come alive again. I wanted to say no, coz I didn't want her to be disappointed that God didn't hear her prayer, but I also wanted to encourage her to believe that prayer is important and powerful. So she placed her little hand on my big tummy and prayed in the simple way that four-year-olds do. And I'm holding onto that prayer. God hears the prayers of little children. I'm holding on with everything I have.

Donald is sad but seems to be coping OK.

My lovely boss came to visit us earlier. I sobbed. I was telling him that I'm dreading labour. I really am. I've done it three times and it's so painful and horrible, but at least you see a living baby at the end of it. I DONT WANT TO PUSH A DEAD BABY OUT!

### Sunday, 16 September 2018

I'm at the hospital now. I've just eaten some Nando's that Donald ordered. We joked around a little. But really, what is there to laugh about? I'm in hospital about to deliver my baby . . . dead.

The room is lovely. The staff seem lovely too. There is a butterfly on the outside of my door, signifying to staff that someone is in there delivering a dead baby. I should stop using the word 'dead'. It feels cold, but to be honest, that's kinda how I feel.

Still holding onto Monique's prayer, I asked the doctor if she could do another scan and double check . . . coz doctors are sometimes wrong, and prayers can be answered. I did feel a bit stupid asking her, but she was lovely and reassured me that it wasn't a stupid request. She performed the scan and just looked at me with sadness. It was true. My baby had died.

I'm tired. It's after midnight now and I think they will be inducing me soon. I'd rather my baby just stayed inside me and somehow seeped back into my skin and blood. The medics did tell me that I didn't have to be induced so soon, I could wait a few more days if I wanted to hold onto my baby that little bit longer, but to be honest I just wanted it over and done with. How could I walk around for a week, looking pregnant, with people making happy comments, knowing the baby inside of me had died? That would have been too odd and too painful.

The midwife has told me that I can administer morphine to myself as and when I feel the need, because they don't want me to feel more labour pain than I need to. I have been dreading this moment, but I do feel a real sense of calm right now. I've been praying. I've been praying a lot. Thank you, God, for peace and calm.

See you on the other side.

## Monday, 17 September 2018

What a day. What. A. Day. I delivered a perfect little baby boy in the early hours of the morning. To my surprise, it was actually really peaceful. The lights were dimmed, it was very quiet, and the midwives popped in and out periodically to see how I was progressing with labour. I was clicking that morphine button like it was going out of fashion, but I could still feel pain.

Donald slept pretty much throughout my entire labour, and to be honest, I'm glad. He is THE most supportive man, but I just felt it would be better for him to be sleeping peacefully rather than watching me going through pain that wasn't going to end well.

When the contractions started to speed up a notch and the pain became more intense, I decided to call the midwife to give me more pain relief. I delivered my other three children without any pain relief, not even gas and air. But this time, I was all for *all* the pain relief. A midwife came to give me some paracetamol. I would have laughed if the pain, physically and emotionally, hadn't been so much. Paracetamol is for a headache, not labour! But before she could even give it to me, I felt the urge to push. I called for Donald to wake up, as I thought he ought to be awake for this bit (dead or alive, this would still be quite a moment for us and our baby) and then I gave one big push. And with that, my baby came out, still enveloped in the amniotic sac, so I was told.

I chose not to look. I didn't know what I was going to see. I didn't know if my baby would look like a baby or not. What if my baby was falling apart coz he had been dead for a while? They asked me if I would like to see him, and I just calmly said no.

I felt relieved that labour was over (coz who enjoys labour pains?) and that it had actually been mentally manageable. I thank God for that because I was really dreading it. The midwives were FANTASTIC. I have never been in a situation like this before, so I had no idea what to expect, but they put absolutely no pressure on me to do, say or feel anything in particular. Although I had chosen not to see my baby, I could hear and see the midwives out of the corner of my eye being so gentle with him and taking care of him as though he was alive. It was beautiful.

I lost all track of time but after a while I told the midwives that I was ready to see my baby. I was far too intrigued not to. But at the same time, I knew that whatever I did see would be the image that would stay in my mind for the rest of my life . . . so I really prayed it would be a nice image.

They wheeled over our baby in a small cot-like bed, but the main difference from a normal baby bed is that this one had a freezing-cold 'mattress' to preserve the appearance of the dead baby for as long as possible. At first, I peered out of the corner of my eye, trying to check that I wasn't going to see something traumatic, and when all seemed fine, I turned my head to have a proper look.

He was gorgeous. So precious and so small. He resembled Gabriel, particularly his mouth. And in his mouth, I could see his little tongue. I marvelled at all the detail of an eighteen-week-old baby from the womb. His face, his fingers, his tummy . . . he even had one of those little clamps on his umbilical cord. Quite simply, he just looked like a very peaceful and ordinary baby. I know people still abort babies in the UK up to twenty-four weeks, so perhaps because of that I assumed that what I would see wouldn't quite be baby-like . . . but nope, this was 100 per cent a fully formed baby with everything in the right place. My baby, who we now decided to name Angelo.

The midwives told us that there was absolutely no rush to leave hospital and that there was a special suite for us and the baby to stay in, with our own little kitchenette so we could just 'live' together for the coming days. As nice an idea as that was, we had three young kids at home and we didn't want to drag out this process any longer than necessary, so we told them thank you but no thank you. But I did want to hold him. He just about fitted in the palm of my hand. What a precious moment. We took pictures. It felt odd to smile in the pictures, so I just tried to look thoughtful.

Always with respect and our permission, the midwives

dressed our baby, took photos and prints of his hands and feet for us and placed him in a little white box with a teddy and keyring. They gave us a matching teddy and the other half of the key ring. A beautiful touch.

Saying goodbye was a weird moment, but I did feel ready. Donald and I prayed today that God would help us use this experience for good. It was so hard to get our heads around what has happened and why ultimately we've just had to 'let go and let God', and I hope this will help to bring us peace and closure.

I'm back home now. As usual, I'm writing now that the kids are in bed. When we got home it was back to parenting three young children, almost like the past twenty-four hours hadn't happened! I'm somewhat grateful for that distraction. I can't imagine the pain of going through that and then coming home to an empty house.

The care, love and attention that my baby received has made all the difference for me today. Honestly, I cannot fault the staff and all they did to honour Angelo.

## Tuesday, 18 September 2018

I woke up and went into autopilot. Back to routine. I got the kids up and dressed and decided to take them to the usual playgroup that we go to on a Tuesday. My mum, who was staying to help, looked at me like I had lost my mind, but I could also tell from her expression that she didn't want to stop me, coz maybe that was my way of coping. So, she got up and said, 'I'll come with you.' I tried to get Donald to come but he was much less willing. He just wanted to clear his head and go for a long bike ride. He hasn't spoken that much. If you dwell on things it doesn't help, does it? I'm not gonna dwell. What's happened has happened. Life continues.

At the playgroup, there were the usual conversations.

'Good weekend?'

I managed to give vague 'it was busy/alright/nothing special' answers. Fortunately, no one there knew I was pregnant. I could see my mum out of the corner of my eye whenever these questions cropped up. I bet she wondered how I was going to respond. She never intervened but it was nice knowing she was there. She's gone home now. I told her I'm fine. Which I am.

Friends are slowly finding out. Some from me. Some from others. Such varied reactions. Obviously, everyone is extremely shocked and sorry to hear what has happened, but you can tell the ones who feel awkward and don't really know what to say, and those who seem more forthcoming with comfort and help. I don't really know what I need, but I'm glad when friends seem like they want to hear more about Angelo. You know that urge you get to bombard friends (and sometimes strangers!) with pictures of your newborn? Well, I still felt that urge. Angelo was in my hands just yesterday and was the most beautiful baby. I still want everyone to see him. My baby. But I've had to stop myself, because who wants to see a photo of a dead baby?

I wonder when he was last alive. I was meant to have a midwife appointment a week sooner than I did but I was busy taking Monique to a shoot for an advert, which was obviously very exciting for us: her first ad. And seeing that this was just a routine appointment *and* it was my fourth child (making me an expert), I felt it was OK to cancel it.

Could that be the single biggest mistake of my life? Maybe when they listened for the heartbeat, they would have picked up a problem and been able to do something about it. Is it my fault that our baby is dead? How was I to know? Everything seemed fine!

We have opted for a post-mortem to be done on Angelo, so we can find out the cause of his death. We won't get the results for three months, though!

I need to sleep. Goodnight.

*Thursday, 20 September 2018*

I've been so wrapped up in thoughts of Angelo that I almost forgot we're in the middle of buying a house. We're relocating out of London and today we had a meeting with our solicitor two hours away to sign the final papers. Donald decided to go to the meeting in shorts. I was so annoyed. Who turns up to a meeting like this in shorts? And then he got annoyed at me for getting annoyed about something so meaningless. We didn't really have much to say to each other for most of the journey. I wish he'd just snap out of it and be normal. I get that he's upset, but he's really dragging the mood down.

*Wednesday, 26 September 2018*

Today would have been my twenty-week scan. To take my mind off it, I decided to take the kids and visit a friend. Once again, Donald decided to stay behind. He's still not saying much about his feelings and I guess we are skirting round the topic a bit, but wallowing in self-pity never helped anyone. He seemed a bit different as we said bye. Anyway, I'm sure he enjoyed the peace and quiet.

My friend was great. We talked and talked. And she gave

me room to do so. And the kids enjoyed playing together. Gabriel fell and cut his lip. It sent shivers down my spine, and it felt like my heart hurt. Ever since Angelo died, I have noticed that I've become very sensitive to my kids' physical pain. And quite protective. I don't really want them out of my sight. I wasn't able to keep a baby alive inside me and how much harder is it to protect children in this big old world? I do think I'm doing OK, though. I've always been quite resilient.

My belly is still big. It's so annoying. I have a big belly and nothing to show for it. And no baby to breastfeed to help bring it down. Last week when my milk came in, that was horrible. The pain of full breasts and no baby to feed. I had to go and buy pads. I felt so stupid. I was worried about someone striking up casual conversation about babies in the aisle. I feel strong enough to talk about it on my own terms, but not at random like that.

Goodnight, diary – I'm tired.

### Saturday, 29 September 2018

I went back to work today. I was on air. Straight back in at the deep end. No support. It was like work were clueless as to what I had just been through. I know I put on a brave face and voice for my listeners, but I'm still human. I'm pleased there weren't many people in the office, though.

Nanite, diary.

### Thursday, 18 October 2018

It was so hard to concentrate at work. When I came off air I found myself desperately wanting to speak to someone who understood what I had been through. Then I got a call. It was the hospital. They said that Angelo's body had been returned following the post-mortem and that we can now proceed with the funeral.

I am dreading it. I genuinely can't imagine how I will make it through. I might just jump in the grave too. I know I put on a brave front, and I've learnt to just crack on with life, but the thought of burying my baby is beyond heartbreaking.

I used to know this lady, briefly, about four years ago, and I remember her talking about her baby who died in the womb. It's been years since we spoke and it's not like we were close, but in that desperate moment today I just needed to reach out. I searched through my phone, found her number, and gave her a call. And what a refreshing call it was. I explained all that had happened, all my anxieties and all my uncertainties, and she just got it. I hope I'm not going to end up annoying her, but I feel like I'm going to latch onto her. She understands. Most people don't seem to.

## Sunday, 28 October 2018

Tomorrow is Angelo's funeral. We've decided to invite close family and friends. We're gonna have a full Mass, go to the cemetery, and then have a little reception back at ours. The madness is, the day after tomorrow is moving day. We are finally moving to our new home. Buying a house and dealing with this, all at the same time, has been A LOT! I feel quite on top of things, although I am constantly wondering whether I will make it through the funeral. I'm dreading tomorrow but at the same time I want it to hurry up and be over with.

I do wonder whether I really am coping alright, which I feel I am, or repressing my true feelings. But what I do know is the power of prayer. I have been praying . . . a lot. Not in a formal way but just conversations with God in my head. Asking Him to give me strength, guidance, wisdom, grace, PEACE! And I believe He is and that's why I'm coping. It doesn't mean that suddenly everything is fine, but it means that when I am vulnerable and lean on Him, He comforts me and gives me the ability to continue.

Donald and I also seem to be connecting properly again. Less surface-level chat. And intimacy has come back too. Part of me wants to get pregnant again quickly. I feel physically empty without my baby. There's meant to be a baby in my tummy. If I conceive now, my baby can still just about make it into the same school year Angelo was meant to be in, with all my friends' kids who are soon to be born. Wouldn't that be great? Otherwise I'm always going to look at their kids and think about what could have been. This wouldn't be replacing Angelo, but just picking up where we left off, right?

Anyway, I've got a bit more packing to do before I sleep. Night.

*Monday, 29 October 2018*

I survived! And I didn't throw myself in the grave! The funeral was nice. I was quite composed until I saw the beautiful, tiny white coffin come out of the back of the funeral car. I was so overcome with emotion. I started to cry, and I remember my priest coming over to me and saying, 'It's OK,' and then I just stopped. Donald carried the coffin in, and the kids followed. They love their brother and, even though they are young, have a beautiful understanding of what is happening. We told them that Angelo died and has gone to be with God in heaven. But only the soul, not the body, goes to heaven, therefore we will bury his body in a safe place. Most days they do talk to me about Angelo. We've always wanted to have quite an honest relationship with the kids, so we've never tiptoed around the subject and have found that children simply understand. They don't overthink things like we adults do.

I couldn't take my eyes off the coffin throughout the service. I kept wondering what Angelo's body looked like now. Not great I imagine. But I was comforted by the fact that he was lying inside a beautiful pouch that my good friend made for him, with his name embroidered on it.

By the time we got to the cemetery it was raining quite a lot, so my mum decided she would take the kids home and wait for us. I really wanted them present. Perhaps it was better than them standing in the rain, but I also wonder if Mum's decision was a cultural thing. I'm pretty sure there is something in the Ghanaian culture about not taking kids to see the burial. I dunno. Anyway, whatever the reason, they missed that bit.

In the end, the urge to jump into the grave wasn't there. Nor did I shed a tear, which surprised me. Each person present threw a bit of soil over the coffin and we said some prayers and then finished. Having this kind of closure was good. As much as I was dreading it, today has been a good day. It reminded me of how much I was dreading the birth and how it turned out to be OK. I'm not saying that any of this is actually fine, but sometimes we can obsess over something in our heads and anticipate the *absolute* worst, when actually, it's bad but not tooooo bad.

Thank you, God, for strength and grace.

Tomorrow, we leave London. A new start!

## Monday, 24 December 2018

It's Christmas Eve! A day when most people are anticipating a fantastic Christmas, but we spent it anticipating Angelo's post-mortem. I can't believe how long it takes to get the results. We asked a couple of friends if they could look after the kids today, as we needed to travel quite a distance back to London to chat to the consultant and get the results. I felt bad coz it's Christmas Eve and people normally have last-minute things to be getting on with, but they were more than happy to help. That's what friends are for :)

We literally had no idea what to expect from the meeting. And I really hoped that nothing was going to show up in the results that indicated that something I had done had caused Angelo's death. I have no idea what that could have been, but the thought can still haunt you. I have spent the last few months wondering whether a urine infection can kill (I often get this in pregnancy), whether ABO incompatibility can kill (that's when the baby's blood type and the mother's blood type are not compatible, causing the baby's red blood cells to break down too much – Emmanuel was born with this and could have been left brain damaged if the problem wasn't spotted and treated so quickly) or whether not taking enough vitamins can kill (I'm rubbish at remembering to take them). At least today we got the answers.

The biggest shock wasn't the result of the post-mortem, it was something else!

So firstly, there was no indication of what made Angelo

die. All organs and blood were functioning normally, and it appears that his heart simply stopped beating. The consult-ant said that in the future, when technology is better, they may be able to find out what caused that to happen, but right now it just looks like an anomaly. That provided a bit of comfort because at least it means the chances of it happening again are slim, but on the other hand it sounds so random that it could happen to anyone, anytime, which is slightly disconcerting.

But like I said, that wasn't the most poignant thing to come out of the meeting. What we did find out was that our darling boy was actually a darling girl! I couldn't believe my ears and what I was reading on the sheet. Of course, she had always been a girl, but the midwife told me the wrong sex when I gave birth. I didn't see a willy, but the midwife said that it just hadn't developed yet. And because I didn't know any better, I just believed her. Now I've been told that the male genitalia would have been present by eighteen weeks and the reason I couldn't see it was because our baby was female!

All over the post-mortem document it was written, 'female', 'female chromosomes'. I was stunned! But also incredibly saddened. Because not only had we named and grieved and buried a baby boy, but in my heart, for the fourth pregnancy, I had realllllllly wanted a girl. So now I'm so con-fused. I don't want to be more upset – whether it was a baby boy or a baby girl, that was still my baby. But at the same time, I'm so so sad that it was my girl after all. I really don't want to start grieving all over again, though. It has taken me three months to get to this place of real peace, so I think the best thing to do is just not dwell on it, park it at the back of my mind, and crack on with Christmas.

*Thursday, 14 February 2019*

It's Valentine's Day today. Not a day that I'm usually bothered about, as Donald and I aren't very sentimental. (My issue, not his.) But today has been weighing heavy on my heart because it was the day our baby was due to be born. Every single Valentine's Day will be tainted by this now. We decided that we would go and visit the grave for the first time since the burial. It would also be the first time seeing the plaque that the funeral directors have erected, which would obviously say 'Angelo'.

I've found it hard over the past couple of months to address the issue that our baby was actually a girl, and because of that we still call her Angelo. Changing the name to a female name would just make it all too real. But in the car today, when we were on our way to the cemetery, we started talking about alternative female names. The obvious choice had been Angela, but I wasn't overly keen on the name. We thought of variations like Angelina, Angelica and Angelique, but none were doing it for me. As I have done throughout the past few months, I continued to speak to God and seek His help and guidance.

Anyway, we reached the cemetery, me, Donald and the three kids, and started looking for Angelo's grave. There were a lot more baby graves there now :(

And then I spotted it. And immediately burst out laughing. The funeral directors had made a mistake on the engraving. Instead of writing Angelo, they had written Angela. Although this wasn't the name I was keen on, I immediately felt peace knowing that God had orchestrated it this way. I hadn't wanted to call the funeral directors to tell them about a name change because I felt so stupid. I had been dreading the emotional decision of picking a girl's name. And then God just went and did it for me. The midwife's error was corrected by the funeral director's error.

Our baby girl, Angela. I felt a real healing instantly. I'm going to be OK. Donald didn't see the funny side of it as quickly as I did, but he too has now come round to it, and has embraced Angela.

*Tuesday, 18 June 2019*

I'm PREGNANT! We're both very happy about this, but I can tell already that there is a tinge of apprehension. Bring on the twelve-week scan. Bring on forty weeks! I've only just found out, but I want to fast forward to the end already.

*Wednesday, 25 Sept 2019*

The anxiety is getting a lot. What if my baby has died? It was at eighteen weeks that I found out that Angela had died, and I'm eighteen weeks now. I've changed GP surgery coz the midwife really didn't seem to care; I've complained to the manager. Nobody at the hospital seems to care either and they are making no effort to give me additional scans or appointments. I don't get it. I'm not attention-seeking; I just want to ensure that the same thing that happened last time doesn't happen again. Why aren't they listening to me? As Black women, we always have to fight harder to be heard and to be taken seriously, but this is horrible.

Anyway, I called the midwife today and just cried down the phone. I begged for a scan, just to put my mind at ease.

She wasn't able to schedule a scan in quickly but she was lovely and told me to come in so she could listen to the heartbeat. And there it was, strong. The relief was immense! But I still felt a level of uncertainty because I'm very aware now that a baby in the womb can die at any time for no apparent reason. I'm trying not to hold on to that though and instead cling to the fact that I heard the heartbeat. As soon as I start feeling regular movement, I know I will relax more. Bring on the movement!

### Friday, 11 October 2019

Hi diary, it's starting to happen. Remember I said that Donald and I prayed that God would use our loss for good? Well, it's happening. Today, I was interviewed on Channel 5 News about breaking the taboo of baby loss! It felt so good to talk. I was extremely ignorant about baby loss until I encountered it, but I've now realised how common it is, starting with the fact that one in four pregnancies ends in miscarriage! Conversations need to be happening at home, in the workplace, with friends, in the government. Baby loss is something awful that far too many suffer silently.

Lord, please continue to use me to break the taboo, but give me the strength and grace to be able to do it. Thank you. Amen.

### Thursday, 5 March 2020

He's here! And what an entrance into the world it was. I'm shattered, so won't write much but Malachi was born late last night after a super-fast and super-intense labour. All glory to God. He is well. I am well. We are home.

*Thursday, 15 October 2020*

I genuinely can't believe what I heard today. I'm trying not to be selfish and make it about me, but would he really have done that to me?

Diary, do you remember back in late September 2018 when I wrote that it would have been my twenty-week scan with Angela, and as I was leaving the house to visit a friend, Donald was acting a bit strange? Well today I found out, by listening to him on a podcast, that he was intending to take his life whilst we were out! WHAT?!

I don't know what to say. I remember that day so vividly. But why? Apparently, he wasn't coping with the recent loss of Angela and had nowhere to turn. He couldn't even turn to me because I was too busy telling him, 'Chin up!' I feel awful. He wrote a letter, left it for me to find, went to 'do it', but lost the nerve at the last moment. Thank God! I'm feeling all kinds of emotions. Some compassion and some anger, and lots of confusion. He didn't realise that I was going to be finding out for the first time when I listened to the podcast. Yes, he had told me in the past that some time ago he had felt suicidal, but I didn't know that it was all planned!

He's now really passionate about men having a safe space to talk honestly about their feelings and what they're going through. It's gonna take me some time to get over this. I know I sound selfish . . . but maybe I am. I will be keeping a closer eye on him, though, and making more of an effort to allow him to cope and process things in the way that works for him. Not what just suits me.

Donald, I'm sorry.

*Tuesday, 19 July 2022*

Today is hot hot HOT and I'm hiding from the sun, coz I'm tired. My body is aching with this baby. I can't believe I'll have five kids soon! I always struggle, not knowing what to say when people say things like, 'Wow, your fifth pregnancy!' or, 'Poor you, one girl and you're gonna have four boys!' Firstly, what gives you the right to make judgements on my household, and secondly, I DID have another girl, but she died!

I'm in such a good place now mentally and emotionally, so I'm able to deal with stupid comments like this, but I do always have to make a judgement call about when to speak my truth and when to just brush it off and walk on by. What I will say is this: children are a real blessing from God. That doesn't mean that if you struggle to have a baby you are not blessed, but it does mean that whether that baby arrived or went straight to heaven, whether it be your first or your tenth, you hold that blessing in your heart forever.

It may be painful, but I know that that blessing has, and will have, a beautiful impact on you in a way you couldn't imagine . . . if you let it.

*Nana-Adwoa Mbeutcha is a home-educating mother of five, a radio producer, and presenter and co-founder of Black Mums Upfront.*

# Loss as a Superpower

*Tom Wateracre*

I think if someone had sat me down in July 2016 and said, 'Your feelings aren't useful or not useful, they're just what you feel,' it would have saved everyone an awful lot of time.

But I am a boy, and a stubborn boy at that, so I decided that my feelings weren't useful, ignored them for two years, and then was really quite debilitatingly sad, and had to pick up the pieces after that.

So that was mistake number one.

Sarah and I had been married for about four years when we had The Talk About Kids. We'd vaguely discussed having children in the marriage preparation course we'd taken because we love drinking bad coffee in church halls, and we'd both expressed ambivalence towards the whole idea. But by the fourth year of our marriage, our body clocks had decided we were a bit more amenable.

Even that was a bit half-hearted, to be honest.

'Shall we just stop using contraception?'

'Yeah, I guess so.'

I suppose we were curious. What might happen here then, eh?

When Sarah became pregnant after about six months, several things suddenly became pretty clear. One: I was thirty-six and Sarah was forty. We went to the hospital for our first midwife appointment, and as the midwife took various data points on her computer, she got to the screen that read 'Is this a geriatric pregnancy?' – a pregnancy where the mother is older than thirty-five. The midwife didn't even ask us the question, just quietly ticked the 'yes' box and moved on, hoping we didn't notice. It felt immediately like the odds were against us.

Two: As we're both practical people, and we like to trade a little in what cognitive behavioural therapy calls 'catastrophising' – anticipating the worst possible outcome as a technique for self-preservation – we decided that our mantra for the pregnancy would be 'hold it lightly'. It's early days, it might not happen, we're older parents, we know the odds are against us – hold it lightly.

Three: As we moved from the twelve-week scan to the fourteen-week scan, we noticed that more and more medical professionals started getting involved. *Uh-oh*, we thought. *Hold it lightly.*

Our baby had a life-limiting genetic condition, a malformed heart, and a single umbilical artery. In combination, the likelihood of our child making it to birth was extremely low, and the likelihood of surviving the birth process or having any kind of quality of life afterwards was even lower. We were offered, and we accepted, a termination at week seventeen.

Throughout the short pregnancy, I had felt the imbalance

in the roles and responsibilities of the different partners quite keenly. Sarah, the person going through the physical pregnancy, needed support, care, attention, which I had to provide. I felt that for me to demand some of the same would be needy. Selfish, even.

When Sarah's pregnancy ended, Sarah – the one who had suffered physical loss, medical intervention – needed support, care and attention. For me to require support, care and attention, well . . . I was holding it lightly, remember?

Sarah had experience of therapy, and almost immediately sought support. We also had one session of couples therapy, which ground to a halt somewhat when I got shirty about the suggestion that we somehow commemorate this significant passing.

'Like, a funeral?' I said. The idea seemed absurd. It was a seventeen-week-old foetus. They didn't have a name. We didn't know – hadn't chosen to know, perhaps – the gender.

I didn't seek my own therapy. I was relentlessly optimistic that we'd get pregnant again quickly. After all, it had only been six months from stopping contraception to this whole business; it was bound to happen again.

As the weeks and months passed, as the near misses and early miscarriages came and went, just a little shade of doubt fell over me. Will this ever actually happen? We had fertility investigations, which came back with no complications ('For your ages,' muttered the fertility doctor.) We focused on the task as if it was something we could control, something rational and fair, which it isn't, of course.

I had quit a well-paid job in a rush and taken a more meaningful role in a charity, trying to get my house in order before the inevitable second pregnancy. But the second pregnancy never came, the meaningful role was stressful, and my mind was elsewhere. Sarah also went through employment miseries – two extremely stressful jobs with badly behaved artists – so I felt pressure to stick with my charity job, but I was getting to the point where I couldn't do that. I needed to be supportive, useful – that was all I felt I was good for in this phase of my life.

I finally broke. I had a panic attack on the train to work, clutching desperately at a handrail to stop myself from falling to the ground, and for the twenty minutes it takes to reach Cannon Street station, I clung there, sweating profusely, feeling like I might die, feeling like I might be dying, feeling like dying might not actually be such an awfully bad thing under the circumstances.

'Your feelings aren't useful or not useful, they're just what you feel.' I quit my charity job and started therapy, and my owl-faced therapist told me that. And after twelve sessions I pretty much believed it. My grief for a seventeen-week-old foetus might have seemed ridiculous to my rational brain, it might have been extremely inconvenient when trying to do basic marketing tasks for a charity, and it definitely wasn't useful – but it was real, and it was what I felt. That baby was a baby I had desperately wanted, it turned out.

My owl-faced therapist also told me I had womb envy, but there didn't seem to be much I could do about that.

So, what were our options? We continued trying for a baby, but after two years of not much success, we were more realistic about the possibilities of conceiving naturally. We had ruled out IVF, as neither of us wanted any more medical intervention for the time being. So that left adoption.

Some friends of ours had adopted, so we knew that, in principle, adoption agencies weren't completely against the idea of comedy writers adopting children. We went to an information evening where some excellent and terrifying social workers did their best to put off anyone entering the process lightly.

I suppose we were curious. What might happen here then, eh?

It took us two years of extra volunteering with children, reading and research, and a little bit more couples therapy to feel in the right place to start the process. After which, we had about six months of training, talking things over with our designated social worker, and – I wish I could give better news on this front – really quite intense investigation of every part of our lives. Seriously, if anyone ever wants to blackmail us, there is a sixty-page document that was written about us that would really help.

Occasionally, I would rant and rave about the process. Our friends didn't have to go through this to have children! They didn't have savings, or spare rooms! They wouldn't be willing to disclose every element of their childhood trauma! Some of them were idiots, or worse, stand-up comedians!

And all the reading around adoption can be tough. The trauma of parental separation upon children is huge, and there are as many complicating factors as there are cases: neglect, abuse, the impact of drugs and alcohol, mental health . . . sad, tough stories. Case studies would often be over a thousand words about the difficulties and sadnesses of parenting followed by the words 'but of course it was the best thing I've ever done', and I'd yell at the book, 'WHY? It sounds so hard! Where are the positives of this whole thing? It's not faaaaair.'

Which it isn't, of course.

But after six months of training and talking and handing over our bank statements and reading detailed paragraphs about why each of our previous relationships had failed, we were approved for adoption, and early permanence.

Ah yes, what's early permanence? They had introduced the concept in the first information evening. While the legal part of adoption is being decided by the courts, adopters are approved as foster carers and look after the children temporarily. If the court rules that separation is best for the child, the approved adopters then step up and adopt their foster placement, reducing the number of times the child has to move from place to place in the care system. If the court rules that the child is safe to return to their birth parents, or extended family, then the approved adopters hand the child back.

It's the 'hand the child back' bit that most people have a problem with.

The social workers at the information evening said that early permanence is primarily for children aged nought to two – some even come directly from the labour ward to the approved adopters' houses. But early permanence is rare, you have to do extra training, and it's not for everyone.

We couldn't fathom who would put themselves forward for this. The risks to the adoptive parents are so high, particularly for people who have already suffered loss and grief.

So, when the time came to tick a box on a form that said 'Are you interested in finding out more about early permanence?', well . . .

I suppose we were curious. What might happen here then, eh?

Throughout the training, a nagging thought started creeping in. Oh no, we thought, what if we're the people who choose early permanence? Part of that was feeling like previous loss might be a superpower. Having been through a cycle of grief, wouldn't we do things differently if it were to happen again? Wouldn't we seek support immediately, and be kind to ourselves, and lean on those around us who will give us strength and sympathy and love?

Smash cut to C – a one-month-and-one-day-old girl – being delivered to our flat by her social worker.

Right then.

I don't want to be cavalier about this or give false hope. Adoption is completely different from case to case, from adopter to adopter. It can be exceptionally sad. It can be really, really difficult. The process can start and stop, speed up, jerk to a halt unexpectedly. Some people find it too much, and I love those people and I understand completely.

As I write, we're waiting for the court to decide whether C will return to her birth family or stay with us. Maybe the court case will happen in September, they say. Or January. It's like that.

Now she's here, what would I say if I were writing a case study, like the ones I had railed against? What are the positives I was looking for?

I can say that every time she stares me directly in the eyes and then deliberately farts, I laugh out loud. I can say that her discoveries – my hands can do this, I can reach that if I really stretch, this tastes surprising – I celebrate with my whole being, right down in my tummy, as though they were my discoveries. I can say that I'm curious to find out if she ever plays the drums, or what kinds of cake she prefers, or if she'll laugh and cry at the same bits of *Paddington 2* as me, or if her flat, flat head ever rounds out.

I can say that, if she goes back to her birth family, as she still could at this point, it will be so sad.

If that happens, we will have to remind ourselves again that what we're feeling might not feel useful, but it will be what we're feeling. That our previous loss and grief can be a superpower. That we should acknowledge what we're feeling, and live in it – and that one day, it will feel less raw.

*Tom Wateracre is a comedian, writer and performer. As a performer, he performed at three Edinburgh Fringes, as well as Latitude, Secret Garden Party and Greenbelt festivals, often alongside his sketch group Pegabovine. As a writer, his work has appeared on BBC Radio 4 and BBC Radio 4 Extra. He lives in London.*

# The Baby-Loss Diaries

### Donald Mbeutcha

### *Friday, 14 September 2018*

What a day. Where do I even begin? I am at work getting on with my day as I normally do. I have meetings
all day, but I have that Friday feeling. My mother-in-law –
who is such a godsend to us – went home last night. So
tonight I can walk around butt naked! I can even fart and not
have to hold it in!

I get a call from Nana-Adwoa mid-morning telling me her
hernia is hurting really bad. My wife being my wife, she is
more worried about the kids being bored than she is about
herself. I tell her they will be fine if they don't do anything
today; you just sit on the sofa and rest. A few hours later she
calls again and, knowing she has a midwife appointment, I
decide to finish up and head home. Meetings will have to
wait till Monday.

As I get home she is feeling better and heading out to her
appointment. I tell her I will come and she says, in classic
Nana-Adwoa style, what about the kids? I say, well, they will
come too! She rolls her eyes and we get in the car. You see, I

don't like to shelter our kids from what we do. I always have this philosophy that we roll as a crew; we either all come, or no one goes.

We are all excited to hear baby's heartbeat. It should sound like a galloping horse, I say to Monique, and make the galloping horse sound. She looks at me and laughs, thinking, *Daddy is silly!*

The midwife then tells us she can't find the heartbeat. It could be baby hiding; it's normal to struggle to find it, she says. If we would like to hear it, she can go and get another, more experienced midwife to try. I leap up straight away and say yes, I would like to hear it, and so would my daughter! The other midwife doesn't have much luck but asks if we would like to hear it at the next appointment or go to the hospital for them to do a scan, as they have more specialist equipment there.

At this point I am concerned, but not thinking the worst. We get to the hospital and they take us to a room. The first doctor walks in, does a check, and walks out again, telling us she needs a second opinion. Another doctor walks in and does the same thing. The third doctor just sits down whilst we have the kids in the room and tells us the news we did not want to hear. There is no heartbeat. Your baby is dead.

What do you mean? How? When? Are you sure? Is this a sick joke? Tears streaming down my face, I look at Nana-Adwoa and she is in bits. A nurse comes in and asks the kids if they want to come with her and do some colouring. I am frozen. I can't . . . I don't know what to do. Where do I start? There is this hole in my heart that has suddenly appeared, but I have no time to think about me or my heart. I can see my wife is in pain, physically and emotionally. I can't add my pain to hers; I need to be there for her. That's my job, right?

Well, she has chosen to give birth to our dead daughter naturally, so we have to go back on Sunday.

Why us, why now?

*Saturday, 15 September 2018*

Did yesterday happen? There was a moment this morning when normality resumed. Kids shouted from their rooms when they were awake, and we woke up and went to see to them. Then this sudden rush of guilt. Why am I smiling – my baby is dead! This rush of it all coming back to me as if I am reliving that moment, over and over again, of the doctor saying, 'Your baby has died.' That is all that is resonating in my head. Nana-Adwoa told me earlier that the doctor could be wrong. My kids have been introduced to death and the eldest is not even five! I keep catching myself having moments of joy and remembering I should be sad because I have lost my baby. I don't know how to deal with this. As a man, I have to put my big-boy mask on and show the world I am OK.

Uncle Muyiwa, my wife's boss, came round to spend some time with us. Whilst he was here, I remembered a wedding I went to in Italy where, as we were getting ready to head to the church, a friend of mine found out that another friend had lost their baby. I remember feeling so sorry for them and not really knowing what to say. Are we now that couple that people will feel sorry for, but not know what to say? I can't even bring myself to pray because I don't think God can understand this one. If He does, why is this happening? What did I do wrong? Is it my fault? Did I not go to the gym enough? Was I not healthy enough? Was my sperm weak? Did I drink too much alcohol?

Snap out of it, Donald – you need to be brave and strong, don't you even dare to cry! Don't be a p****! Man the f*** up! The baby is delivered tomorrow so put on your big-boy pants!

*Sunday, 16 September 2018*

My mother-in-law came last night so we could go into hospital today. Is something wrong with me? Should I have been mourning this whole time? What does it look like to mourn a baby that you have not seen?

We get to the hospital in a strangely good mood. There is an air of excitement. Is that normal? We discuss what is about to happen and I wonder whether she feels hurt like I do. The truth is, I am broken, but I have to be strong, right? I have to be: for her, for the kids, for everyone else.

As we approach reception, we tell them why we are here and it's the first time it hits me. It's like someone has punched me in the face. We are taken to this room which feels so warm yet so cold. As we walk down the ward, we can hear faint screams of mothers giving birth. My mind begins to wonder, are their children alive? Is this a cruel joke where we get put in a room where we can hear women giving birth? I don't even know what to expect with this birth. Our son or daughter will be born dead! Will Nana-Adwoa go through labour – what will that be like? I suddenly feel sick; I need to stop overthinking. NANDO'S! I order some Nando's. The process of getting that on Deliveroo will take my mind off it. I don't want to think about this!

Nana-Adwoa asks me if we should ask the doctor for another scan, just in case they made a mistake. That's a lot of hope to allow ourselves to have, for it to be snatched away if the baby is still dead at the end of it. But it's not about me; it's about her, and I want to make sure I do everything I can for my wife. I put my thoughts to the side and say, of course! Our God is a God of miracles! I am trying to hold onto that and really believe it, but the truth is it's very hard. I feel sort of half-hearted about it. Is that bad? Is it my fault if our baby is still dead because I only half believe? Man, this is tough.

Nana-Adwoa has been induced, so now it's a waiting game. I lie on the sofa in this beautiful room I haven't even had the chance to take in. Nana-Adwoa is lying on the bed. It is really nice; it seems so tranquil. Gosh, what happens next? I say to Nana-Adwoa, 'If you feel anything, let me know.'

I am feeling tired now; my mind hasn't stopped. What do I say to people? What happens next? What about the kids? Imagine how they must be feeling, their little minds.

*Monday, 17 September 2018*

Today our baby boy came. The cry a baby makes when they are born, I waited and waited and waited and it didn't come. I knew it wouldn't, but there was part of me that expected something. I don't know what, but I did.

He was born in the early hours of the morning. The midwives had been coming in and out and I was wakened from the deepest sleep by Nana-Adwoa telling me she needed to push: this was it, the baby was coming. I had never looked down the business end before, I was not about to start now! So, I rushed to hold her hand and with one almighty push and tears streaming down her face, baby was out.

There was a rush of emotion that came with that big push and those words she uttered next: 'Do you want to see?'

Why would I want to see? I am not ready for that! I did not know what to expect but the chance to see my baby, who was dead, was certainly not it.

My heart was pounding; I couldn't stop tearing up. 'I don't want to see,' I said to the midwife. She took our baby away, still in the same room as us but just out of sight.

I think it was my wife who said she was ready to see our baby. They wheeled him over in a cold cot. He just looked like he was asleep, perfectly formed. This was a baby; this was our baby! Can you believe that he was in my wife's body and all he had to do was keep putting on weight?

Our baby was dressed, and we took pictures. Pictures I don't think I will be ready to see for a little while. What happens now – what do we do now? We were handed a pack that has information around miscarriage and stillbirth. Our son's hand and foot imprints were taken. The midwives gave us half a keyring and told us the other half would be with our baby along with a teddy matching the one they gave us. We discussed the autopsy options and what would happen next. I have already had to travel back and forth from home to hospital a few times since being here, which at least has been a distraction from how I am feeling.

*Tuesday, 18 September 2018*

Nana-Adwoa woke up this morning and decided she was just going to get the kids ready and go to a playgroup. Errrmmm, hello lady, you gave birth to a dead baby yesterday! What's wrong with you? We have not even had a chance to talk about it and you are just getting on with life like nothing happened! I am very much like my mum: I want us to talk through things and cry or whatever you do. She asked if I wanted to come with them, but right now I don't even want to see my own kids, let alone other people. 'I am not going out with you,' I say to her, 'I just want to be by myself.' Maybe I'll go out for a bike ride. Outside seems so big. I want my baby boy. I don't want anything else that outside has to offer.

I have been slowly telling people: family members, etc. My boss offered to call but I could not bring myself to speak with him. I don't want to speak to anyone. Someone said that it was just a bunch of cells. Someone else said that we already have three kids and what about those that don't have any? Today feels very sad for me; I feel alone. Have you ever been alone even though there are people around you? That's exactly how I feel. I feel the pressure from my wife to just get on with it, but I can't; I am not built like that. My wife is psychologically stronger than I am.

I sat in our bedroom for a few hours and looked at the memory box they gave us. Just stared at it, couldn't bring myself to open it or look in it. I hope tomorrow is a better day, because I don't feel right.

*Tuesday, 25 September 2018*

Wow! I have not been able to write or articulate how I am feeling. I am in pain emotionally, psychologically, physically. I am hurting. I had a panic attack today. I had to run into our utility room and lock myself in, pretending to be on the toilet just to get my breath back and compose myself.

No one has really asked how I am, how I am feeling. I want to talk to someone, but I get the sense people are avoiding us because they don't know what to say. This is so weird; I am finding out who my friends really are. A lot of them have created a distance so they don't have to speak about it to us. Why are we friends with these people again? I feel so helpless. Over the last week I have blamed myself for everything. I have come to the conclusion that if it wasn't for me, our child would not have died. Now he is alone, not knowing who his mummy and daddy are. I want to hold my baby; I want to be with my baby!

I have googled too many times ways to take my own life so I can be with my baby. Then this hole in my heart, this weight I am carrying will be gone. I have written a letter and I am hoping that when Nana-Adwoa finds it, she will understand why and not be sad. That way, she can take care of our babies here and I will take care of our Angelo. She will explain it to the kids and it will make sense. And if they don't understand, they are like everyone else. They never wanted to understand how I felt. I am not built as strong as my wife.

*Wednesday, 26 September 2018*

Nana-Adwoa went to see her friend with the kids today. I had a few hours, which gave me enough time. I so badly wanted to tell her that I was going to be with our baby, but I couldn't bring myself to. I hugged the kids extra tight; the goodbye was a bit more prolonged than usual. As soon as the door was shut, I fell to my knees, crying uncontrollably. Tears streamed down my face as I said, 'I am coming, Angelo! Hold on, Daddy is coming to be with you so you won't be alone anymore.' I took myself upstairs with a bottle of whisky, pulled out the note I had written yesterday and placed it in the middle of our bed. The stark realisation of what was about to happen filled me with dread and joy at the same time.

On one hand, I thought, I will be with my baby, but on the other, all the things I want to achieve I will no longer be able to do. Walking my daughter down the aisle. Growing old with my wife. But I don't want my baby to be without me; wherever he is, I want to be with him. I don't want anything else but to be with my baby! There is nothing this world can offer me right now. I am tired; no one even cares. No one has even asked me or spoken to me about how I am, so why would they care if I am gone? I want to go and be somewhere better than where I am now and that's with my son.

I cried and cried.

The whisky, let's start with that. As I opened it, I heard the door go and the kids and Nana-Adwoa walk in. I quickly jumped up and put everything away. I have never been so glad to hear my family come home.

A moment of clarity hit me today as I realised that this didn't happen to us by chance. Life is the most precious gift that can be given to any of us and when it's taken away in this way, it must leave a legacy in its trail.

*Saturday, 29 September 2018*

Nana-Adwoa went back to work. What a trialling day it has been. To see the smiles on my children's faces has been a blessing, but I can't help but think that there is one missing. Everything still feels so incomplete. At times, I catch myself feeling sad and returning to thoughts of wanting to be with my son, but I quickly snap out of it. I am still struggling.

How do people do this? I read a story about an MP who has had multiple miscarriages. How does she do it? How does *he* do it? Am I the weak one here, or am I missing something I should be getting?

*Monday, 1 October 2018*

My first day back in the office. All through my journey in I was wishing it would take slightly longer. I was dreading speaking with anyone about it. A few days ago, I got a message from my boss asking me how I would like people to deal with it: talk about it, not talk about it, etc. I just said I was happy to talk about it if it comes up in conversation. Am I, though? Well, it came up a few times. First there was that awkwardness, then a colleague came and gave me a hug. She broke down. I thought to myself, why are you crying? You're not the one who has lost a child. Moreover, don't get your makeup on my shirt, that will not be cool! Anyway, she said she was so sad that it happened to me. That was touching, really. I started to feel part of a community of people who cared somewhat. I also found out that my boss has been through a similar thing. He never spoke about it, but why would he, it's not the ideal topic of conversation when you meet people, is it?

An old colleague reached out to me and mentioned that there is a group of dads that was created a few months back, some of whom have been through the same thing. He said he will add me to the group if I want him to. I agreed. Let's see what happens.

I completely forgot we are trying to move. The solicitor and estate agent called today as well. Great, something else I have to think about!

## Friday, 26 October 2018

Today was tough. We have been planning a funeral for our baby boy for about a week, and today Nana-Adwoa got the call to say that the body was ready to be buried. I asked if we could see him one last time, but we were advised against it. They said it was better we remembered him with the pictures we had. I was going to push and probe, but my heart aches and I could feel those feelings coming back.

We are also moving tomorrow so we have been packing and all sorts. It's a lot!

We had close friends and family come. As I picked up his little coffin to carry him into the church, my heart sank and I started to shake. I could feel my hands getting sweaty and for a moment I was transported to a different place. My mind and thoughts were in overdrive. I should not be carrying this; this is not the order of things. I nearly turned back and ran and didn't complete the walk. We had only told a few friends, so when I glanced up and saw a friend who had come from Manchester to be with us, I felt comforted. You know when you are on the verge of tears, and you get a hug from a person who loves you, and it brings you to more uncontrollable tears but also the warmth of comfort? That was what I felt. We never quite know what impact our actions have, but no matter how small or big, they always have an impact on someone, and that's what she did for us.

I walked down the aisle with the kids behind me, and I felt courage and strength knowing that all my children were finally in one place, together. The ones behind me and the one I was holding. That image is one that I will hold onto forever. It got me thinking about when the right time is to introduce kids to the concept of death. Gosh, we haven't even stopped to talk to them about it! They seem to have an understanding that their brother has gone to an amazing place in spirit, but we will bury his body today. If only we were more like kids, life would be so much simpler.

Anyway, back to the packing. I can feel Nana-Adwoa looking for me already. She is a woman on a mission. We still have so much to do to leave here tomorrow. To new beginnings with, hopefully, healed scars of the past.

## Monday, 24 December 2018

Guess where we are? Back at the hospital where Angelo was born. It has taken a while for what we are about to hear. I have blamed myself many times for him dying. Asked myself a million and one questions. I have even questioned whether Nana-Adwoa did everything she could have done or whether she missed something. Now we get to hear the scientific reason after the autopsy. As the doctor is talking, I keep hearing 'she', 'her', etc., and I stop and ask her, 'What do you mean, her? Have you got the right results?' She says, 'Yeah!' So we buried and mourned a he, and now we have to mourn a her! How does that even make sense? The results, at this point, I can't even take in. I am still trying to comprehend what happened there! How does he turn into her?

I know Nana-Adwoa and our eldest wanted a girl this time, so I think the fact that it was a girl really hit her hard. She showed more emotion when she heard this news than she had before. I really don't even know what to say at this point.

I am tired. All of this has taken a toll on my mind. The move was a nice distraction, but this has all brought back so many memories. Maybe I need to speak to a professional. Do I, though? I am not crazy. What do I say? 'Hi, my name is Donald, and I lost my baby.' That sounds so soft and wet! People will laugh at me. I don't know if I have the courage for that yet.

### Thursday, 14 February 2019

Today was Angela's due date. Over the last few months, I have reached out to a charity called Sands and spoken to counsellors there who deal with parents who have suffered loss. To be honest, they were crap at first, and I had to try several times to get through and speak with someone. I decided to get my own counsellor as well. I have had four sessions so far, and just to have someone to talk to in a place where I will not be judged . . . I can be free! It has been difficult to express all that I am thinking, all I want and all I don't want. I have also started encountering men who have been through a similar thing. One of them lost twins and I have tried to be there for him. Man, this journey is harder than I thought. In fact, I hadn't even thought.

### Saturday, 17 September 2022

Today marks four years since Angela was born dead. Just writing those words hits home what we experienced and makes me relive those emotions again. All day it has been difficult to do anything. The day started off with two of our friends who always remember Angela's birthday. The kids wanted to go to the beach because that's what we did on her first birthday and since then they have seen that as the thing we do. Only this year I wasn't really feeling it. It was the first time I just wanted to be at home with the family, pottering about in the house. I have come a long way when I think about it, and what has kept me going is my faith and the love around me, but also the spaces I have created for other men to feel the same. For them not to fall into what I fell into.

Life has been tough these last few years, especially last year. I was in intensive care twice and nearly died (another story for another day). I just need to remind myself that sometimes all I have to do is create the space for men, dads, anyone to talk, because when it comes down to it, living in our own heads is not what we are designed to do. We all need someone to talk to.

A few weeks ago, the kids found a poem that I wrote for Baby Loss Awareness Week whilst I was learning to walk again in rehab, and were playing it on YouTube. That poem is all about being a father to babies who may not be here with us physically, and knowing that does not make us worse, or less, or not fathers.

*Donald Mbeutcha is a trustee of Beyond Equality and Race Equality Foundation, and head of partnerships at Best of Africa, and was previously part of Dope Black Dads.*

*When life is difficult, Samaritans are here – day or night, 365 days a year. You can call them for free on 116 123, email them at jo@samaritans.org, or visit samaritans.org to find your nearest branch.*

# Living

# Eshet Chayil

*Sarah Lewis*

As far back as I can remember, my mum made chicken soup every Friday night. Nicknamed 'Jewish penicillin', it's supposed to help ease physical ailments and mental anguish and is a staple in most Jewish homes. There is no secret recipe, although you might think so from the way each family tries to guard its own. We see generations of mothers passing down prized chicken-soup recipes to their daughters in the sound knowledge that they, in turn, will do the same.

These days I am a lapsed cultural Jew because, as someone without children, my Judaism has lost much of its meaning. I still enjoy making a soulful Friday-night dinner, but most other things have gradually fallen by the wayside. One of the holiest days in the calendar is Yom Kippur, the day of atonement. Even if you aren't religious, you turn up and ask for forgiveness! Call it Jewish guilt or tradition, either way the synagogues are packed. Part of the service is the confession of sins. There is a line that reads, 'And for the sins for which we incur the penalty of excision and childlessness.' It doesn't take a genius to work out how a childless woman might struggle with that line, and it's not the only place that

Judaism confronts childlessness in this way. I think it's fair to say that Judaism is pronatalism on steroids.

In their most distilled and simple terms, the roles of men and women in the Orthodox tradition of Judaism are easy to understand. Although both sexes were apparently created in the image of God, each has different responsibilities and obligations, which are thought to complement the other. Men were made head of the household, commanded to read from the holy scriptures and ensure the family adhered to a Jewish way of life. Much of the time they would be attending or running religious services, while a woman's responsibilities were largely based at home, with the obligations of being a good wife, bearing children and being the ultimate home-maker. In many households on a Friday night during Shabbat prayers, the man of the house will still sing 'Eshet Chayil' (Woman of Valour) to his wife. It is a song which praises with gratitude the woman of the house for her strength and positive conduct, the management of her home, her community, her husband – and her children.

It still feels almost unthinkable that I am 'Jewish and childless'. Those two words simply don't fit together. Who am I if I don't have children? What place do I have in my community? My identity as a Jewish woman was gone for-ever, making room for the perfect existential crisis. It has been a complex and painful journey from which I thought I might never recover and there have been times when a life without children was one that I simply didn't want. I can say to those on their own childless journey that I have learned that together we are a tribe of survivors with rare insights to bring to this world.

*

With an English mother and Israeli father, our family life in England was traditional and quasi-religious, with a strong Israeli influence. Both sides of my family originated from Eastern Europe. Dad's parents and one of his aunts were the only ones from their family that survived the Holocaust because they fled their homes in 1936. Our family went to synagogue on High Holy Days. My brothers and I had bar and bat mitzvahs respectively, and Mum kept a kosher home. We were part of a thriving Jewish community, and our house was always full of extended family and friends, sitting down for a Shabbat meal. Judaism is steeped in magnificent traditions passed down through the generations – just as Tevye sang about in *Fiddler on the Roof.*

My early childhood was a very happy time. I remember being excitable, courageous and fiercely independent. I went to the local Jewish primary school and spent my free time either sitting barefoot underneath our willow tree and daydreaming, or busy with parentally encouraged extra-curricular activities. I laughed, sang and danced my way to grammar school. The next phase of my life set me on a path away from all that I knew, and to which I would not return until my late thirties. While my friends from primary school seemed happily cocooned at other schools, at mine I was subjected to a torrent of systematic bullying. I was confident and outspoken, and I clearly had 'target' written all over my back. It led me to become withdrawn and rebellious. I flunked school, dropped out of A levels, and then left home.

I fell into my first long-term relationship at nineteen with a man thirteen years older than me. Our worlds collided, and I went dancing with the devil. With no alarm bells ringing, the beginning of my spiritual journey had begun. The naive elation of meeting the man who I thought was my soulmate ended several years later, by which time I was estranged from my family and community, having miscarried my first child. I graduated with nine A-stars from the 'School of Life'.

I was twenty-six when I left town to escape, where I managed to hustle my way into my first 'proper job'. I poured what was left of me into that job, becoming a workaholic and putting the last fifteen years in a mental box for safekeeping. I spent the next ten years climbing the corporate ladder, having to work harder than my degree-educated counterparts. I felt jealous of those who sailed through these years largely unscathed, who looked like they were winning in the game of 'happily ever after'. My contemporaries were now all in top jobs or married stay-at-home mums doing the school run in their 4x4s. If I saw them in the street, I used to cross over to avoid them, desperate not to have to engage in any small talk.

I really wasn't interested in settling down; my rebellious phase lasted a little longer than perhaps it should. I could drink and party till the early hours – and still can if required, although these days I am normally in bed by 11 p.m., catching up on the day's news, and that's just how I like it. I had no idea what a healthy relationship looked like: platonic, romantic or otherwise. There was plenty of collateral damage when people tried their best to help me. Everyone except me knew that the way to heal and mature was through letting people in, not shutting them out.

When I finally bought my first apartment, I was still single so I spent many a Friday night at their house having Shabbat dinner. Not only was it amazing not to have to cook after a long week at work, but it also brought me back to my religion. Listening to my dad reciting the Friday-night prayers always made me feel like I was in the right place, and it still does, because Shabbat is the time to be with family. Spending those evenings with them are some of my fondest memories.

Their friends would constantly ask about my plans for meeting a man. On the one hand I felt that time was ticking, but on the other I was still enjoying a carefree single lifestyle. There can of course be cock-ups with that, and in my mid-thirties I was left having to make the most painful decision when I found myself accidentally pregnant. For many years, and still sometimes if I'm having a bad day, I see my childlessness as payback.

I realised that things had to change. I was youngish with an interesting career, and I thought I was good company. I felt I had a lot to offer the right person, if only I could find him and tackle my commitment-phobia. My husband once joked that at twenty, women want a man who's never been married; at thirty they may consider a divorcé as the pool of eligibles shrinks, and by thirty-seven (when I met him), you'd consider marrying a divorcé with children!

I met him on a Jewish online dating site. How utterly uncool. Being mostly disconnected from anything or anyone Jewish, it was all a little weird, but meeting him was like coming home. He had been divorced for almost two years and, randomly, our parents already knew each other. What were the chances? I tried to play it cool, yet six weeks later we were both firmly committed.

I had been adamant through our initial courtship that I

didn't want children, and he was medically no longer able, so that was that. I moved into his house after a few months. I'd lived alone for many years, and I am someone who loves a quiet house. Are you worried yet? You should be! The children were all under twelve and, without the distraction of having my own children, they had my undivided attention as I threw myself into being a stepmum. I was excelling in my career and within a matter of weeks was also throwing birthday parties, baking novelty cakes, giving lifts and drop-offs here and there and, because I apparently have better fashion sense than their father, I was also shopping for cool teenage outfits. I have heard this type of stepmum behaviour referred to as step-smothering. I don't entirely disagree!

I was lovingly adopted by my husband's community. I finally learned to cook, and our home was always full of friends and family. It all happened very quickly. In hindsight, perhaps too quickly. I raced through the next couple of years juggling a crazy work schedule, constant entertaining, organising our wedding and a bar mitzvah. I was getting good at the wife and stepmum thing. I had surprised myself at how well I had coped – flourished, even – and I loved being part of such a vibrant community. Life started to make sense, and for the first time I felt I belonged. It was then that the feelings of wanting a child of my own suddenly started to creep in. I laughed off the idea at first, knowing that my husband was no longer able to have children, but eventually I was consumed with longing to share a child with him and to create our own family. I have since learned that you can convince yourself of pretty much anything if the will is there. Isn't there a slim chance that science can be wrong? When I skipped two periods, after being regular like clockwork for most of my life, I was convinced, without doubt, that I was pregnant. The test said otherwise, and I cried myself to sleep.

There was little time for us to build our new marriage. Half the time we had kids and the other half we were exhausted. The first signs of resentment were showing on both sides. My husband wondered where his carefree and fun fiancée had disappeared to, and the more deeply rooted I became in the suburban Jewish dream, the more I felt like an outsider. I'd spend hours preparing big Shabbat dinners and festival meals for friends and family, only to feel excluded from the constant conversation about children at my own table. Everywhere, life was full of these little exclusions. I became a master at exiting a room when things became overwhelming. When friends would hear me say I was going to 'get a jumper', they knew that I had taken myself home or off to bed. I am certain most of them never realised the real reason and simply thought my social meter had run out.

I am one of only three childless women in our Jewish community of nearly 300 families, and the only one of my generation. The only other childless woman I knew went on to have a 'miracle baby' in her early forties. Of course she bloody did. Then a few weeks after my husband and I married, I was walking down the road to a party with one of my closest friends when she stopped in the middle of the road and said, 'I need to tell you something.' I could see the sympathy in her eyes before the words rolled out of her mouth. 'I'm pregnant.' For a few long seconds, motherhood crashed down between us until I pushed out an overly loud and excitable congratulations as I wiped a quick tear from my face. She was forty-three and already had two children. She asked if we would be godparents, which felt like a twist of the knife she'd just stabbed me with. I really was truly excited for her and honoured to be asked, but I have learned that you can feel immeasurable joy for others at the same time as shedding tears of personal pain. As we arrived at the party, I grabbed a large cocktail, headed straight into the garden where nobody could see me, and wept. It was on that night that I finally realised I was never going to become a mother. Over the years, my husband and I had discussed and briefly looked into fostering but the complexities of attempting to travel that road within what was an already challenging blended family dynamic made the reality untenable.

I didn't recognise my feelings of resentment as signs of grief until I gave up my job to try and restore some balance. When I stopped working and my world became smaller, my grief got larger and so did I. I piled on twenty-five kilos and was unrecognisable. My time mostly revolved around my husband, the kids and our community. I was often in synagogue helping out with one thing or another, but I started to find it triggering because it is always full of families and young children, so I gradually stopped helping and attending for services.

Everywhere I went, all I could see were families, or mums pushing prams. Even the supermarket shop became overwhelming. It wasn't too long before I completely excluded myself from everything social too. My reserves were diminishing and there was a limit to how many times I could subconsciously hear the same old line of 'P.S. You're not invited'. Whilst my friends were out at their 'parent' friends' parties, I was at home desperately trying to come to terms with the fact that I would never have a little hand to hold in mine, be able to teach my daughter how to say the blessing over the Shabbat candles or have someone to teach the festival songs to. I felt guilt because I hadn't produced offspring to carry on my family line, especially after everything we had overcome in the generations before me. My rescue cat, who had joined our family several years earlier, became my saviour, and it was me and her against the world. She would lovingly curl up in my arms for hours at a time when I was home alone, buried in grief. She was an enormous comfort to me and a legendary companion. I know it was difficult for everyone in my household to live alongside the grieving version of me, whether they understood what was happening at the time or not.

When you long to be a mother, there are so many triggering occasions which you must learn to navigate. I wouldn't say I have navigated any of them particularly gracefully – I try to forgive myself for that. Coping gets easier, but the pain is always there. You learn to build a new life around the grief, so that it becomes a lesser part of you, but the pain will always remain in some form. Part of grieving is ugly and embarrassing, for there is no rule book to guide you. Learning when it is OK to say no to avoid being in certain situations to protect yourself is a matter of trial and error.

My first attempts to find support within my own community were met with advice on fertility clinics and the brutal yet well-meaning idea that barren women automatically get a place next to God in heaven – yes, really. Thank God I found Jody Day's Gateway Women community. The lack of empathy and understanding as to how a Jewish woman might find herself childless was breathtaking. I was grieving a loss that they simply couldn't understand and was struggling with my sense of identity because of it. I was lost and desperate for spiritual guidance to help me make sense of my situation, but instead had to look outside of my community to find it.

I lost years to the grief and, along with it, many friends and almost my marriage too. Humans can be full of complex and conflicting emotions, and whilst I love, admire and respect my husband, sometimes I feel jealous and happy for him at the same time. Other times I wish I could reap the benefits afforded to those without any children at all. It has often felt like living in no-man's land. I don't quite fit in with my parent friends or with my childless friends.

Recovery from grief has been like reinventing myself over and over, and I'm not quite finished yet. I needed new experiences to break me out of the cycle of grief and so I slowly dipped my toe back into the outside world. I felt like a stranger at first. I hadn't been around people for a long time and perhaps I had become a little feral. It felt in many ways like a completely new life, and it took many attempts to push myself out of the door.

Meeting new people and trying new things felt daunting and sometimes it would end in tears or frustration. Occasionally, like an injured animal I would retreat to my bedroom to lick my wounds before trying again. Like many, I crave the feeling of being accepted and finding commonality with others. I have found that many women will open a conversation with 'Have you got children?' as a way of making a quick connection, presuming that the answer will be a yes. Those moments were really tough, as the chance of potential kinship and commonality all but disappeared. It took me several years to navigate them and to dodge the various follow-ups when the well-meaning would proffer suggestions of adoption or fostering as a lifeline. Nowadays when people ask me if I have children, I am learning to just say 'no', then smile and move the conversation on.

Being back in the real world, I finally found that there was promise, opportunity and hope. There were moments where I was overjoyed because I didn't think I would ever feel that again. Little sparks of joy gave me something tangible to build on, so I kept going. Even though good days were dotted amongst griefy days, each time I looked behind me, I felt further away from my very darkest corner.

In the last three years I have studied, set up a business, and tried out various jobs to see what made me light up inside again. I have had to learn how to curate this new life when it comes to friends and family. For those who repeatedly activated my triggers, I have moved in a different direction. For those who have ridden beside me during my very dark moments, including my tribe at Gateway Women, I feel forever indebted. I have largely stayed away from synagogue because the feelings of exclusion and isolation are still difficult to cope with. There has been a price to pay in the fact that I am less connected to my Jewish friends than I would otherwise have been. I hope for future generations that the attitude towards childlessness will change and that modern Orthodoxy will learn to include and value everyone. Part of recovery and moving towards living a fulfilling, adapted, childfree life has been to try and connect with more childless people because we have an unspoken language of support and understanding.

Being a childless stepmum is forever. It is a difficult

journey to navigate, and one which goes unrewarded a lot of the time. I have so much appreciation for those who give selflessly to love and protect children that are not biologically theirs. I have done so freely and without regret. I feel lucky to have an active role in my stepchildren's lives, an opportunity which I might not have had if I hadn't met my husband. I am extremely proud of them and have boundless love for them, even when they don't do what they say on the tin!

I have had the unwavering support of my husband. We are continually learning and growing together as we try to successfully navigate our blended family life. We are a formidable team that has grown stronger and closer through much adversity. We often discuss how wonderful it would've been if we had met each other the first time around, but life can be a messy journey with many unexpected plot twists. My dad always says 'life is like a big dream' and he is right. Time passes so quickly, and we each have a choice whether to give in to the darkness or to walk courageously into the light.

*When I found myself childless, I struggled to find Jewish voices that resonated with my own and it felt very isolating. In order to share my story openly in the hope that it might resonate with you, I have included experiences which involve my immediate family. I hope you will understand that, to protect their privacy, I have chosen to write my essay under a pseudonym.*

# Work in Progress

*Rageshri Dhairyawan*

There's a scene in *Friends* that sticks in my memory. Ross and Rachel are attending their first antenatal ultrasound scan. Rachel is dressed in a blue hospital gown, lying on a bed as Ross points to where the baby is on the screen. She pretends that she's seen it, but he realises she hasn't when she worries that she's a *bad mother* because she can't see her baby. He shows her again and finally, she sees it. They both stare at the screen, hands tightly entwined.

I was twenty-one and at university when this episode came out and had no doubt that this was a moment that I could look forward to sharing with my future partner. With the confidence of youth, I knew that I'd be able to see my baby first time because I was sure I'd be a *good mother*. I couldn't imagine a future where this wasn't even a possibility.

In the end, I did see ultrasound images with my husband, but it was not in a manner I had expected.

Starting our family was proving to be more difficult than we had anticipated. Having come off the contraceptive pill to conceive, I started to suffer from debilitating period pains. After a few months of going back and forth with my GP, I was referred to gynaecology and listed for keyhole surgery to investigate what was going on. I came round from the anaesthetic to be told that I had stage four endometriosis – the most severe – which had damaged my internal organs to such an extent that it was unlikely that we would get pregnant naturally. The gynaecologist advised that we would need IVF. After several operations and hormonal treatment to calm the endometriosis down, we began fertility treatment in 2012, with great hope and expectation.

It was during our third, and then fourth, IVF cycles that we were given photos of the ultrasound scan performed at embryo transfer. Embryos safely tucked inside my womb, we'd be handed photos of what could be our future children and sent home for the two-week wait until we could take a pregnancy test. Unlike antenatal photos, which have the discernible image of something that looks like a baby, the embryos were too small and unfamiliar to see. The only thing that stood out in those grainy black-and-white images was my uterus and the intrusive line of the pipette used to carry the embryos. I'd start each day of those two weeks looking at them, imagining I could see the embryos and wishing that this time our cycle would be successful.

But they never were. None of our four cycles led to a pregnancy, let alone a baby. What remained was these photos as the sole substantial evidence of the potential children that we had created together. Also, a reminder to me that I had failed. I was such a bad mother that the embryos had felt unable to make themselves at home in my body.

It was hard to know what we should do with the images.

Throwing them away felt wrong. But neither could we proudly display them in our home or show them to friends and family. What do you do with photos of something that existed for five days in a petri dish? And how do you grieve their loss? As well as not seeing the embryos on the scan, was there anything else I was finding difficult to see?

Ten years on, these are questions that I am still trying to resolve.

After almost twenty years of working continually full-time as an NHS doctor, I've taken some time out. Working through the Covid-19 pandemic was hard and I needed to pause. I decided to take a year's sabbatical to do a master's degree. I reasoned that this would provide me with the opportunity to learn new skills that would be useful for future research, as well as a break from clinical practice.

I left work at the end of September 2021 and by Christmas I had come to understand that the old adage 'a change is as good as a rest' was not true for me. Whilst I was enjoying the master's, which was challenging my brain in new ways, it was more work than I had expected. I was exhausted and feeling unsettled. I had experienced not only a significant change in my routine, but also a loss of identity. I had gone from feeling useful as a senior doctor treating sick patients to sitting in seminars with fellow students half my age. This was a shock. I thought it was a good time to restart therapy.

During my sessions I noticed that the subject of being childless was increasingly coming up. Away from the stresses and responsibilities of work, space for other feelings was growing, and the sadness of not being a mum was creeping back in. I thought this was something I had dealt with and that I was doing OK, but perhaps this wasn't the case. Instead of ignoring the sadness, suppressing it and moving on, this time I wanted to bring it into the light and examine it.

I remembered how, several years earlier, I'd attended a course for consultants supervising junior doctors working less than full-time. I had never had this experience, so wanted to find out how I could better support my trainees.

The course facilitator had started by presenting reasons for why junior doctors choose to work part-time. She said it was often for caring duties, sometimes for a better work-life balance, occasionally to take time for other projects like training for a marathon. This would have been frowned upon when we were junior doctors, the trainer explained, but was now much more acceptable. I admit, I internally rolled my eyes at this. *Junior doctors have it easy these days*, I found myself thinking, before admonishing myself for sounding like a dinosaur.

But then I heard the words 'fertility treatment'. One of the fellow attendees said they were supervising a trainee who was going part-time for a year to have IVF. How could he support her with this? The facilitator told us that fertility treatment was one of the main reasons female trainees work less than full-time. I was gobsmacked. Just a few years before, I had never realised that was an option for me and had continued to work full-time for the three years we had treatment, fitting appointments around my clinical duties and taking the occasional sick day or annual leave to recover from procedures. Why didn't someone tell me? And even if they had, would I have let myself go for it?

If I am to be truly honest with myself, I know I wouldn't have. I had spent years working in a culture that has traditionally valorised hard work to the detriment of people's personal lives. Going above and beyond your duties in medicine is seen as normal and expected. I've learned to be good at caring for other people. I'm less good at looking after myself.

Nowhere is this more evident to me than when we received the results of our fourth IVF cycle in 2013. We had decided that this was going to be our last, as I had become unwell with previous treatment, and we weren't sure that more could be done to improve our chances of success.

We had done everything we could. To improve the quality of my eggs, I upped my intake of recommended vitamins and minerals; I had overcome my childhood milk phobia by drinking milkshakes flavoured with rose syrup daily; I was eating Brazil nuts and pineapple. I was injecting myself with the drugs, taking the pills, and using the vaginal gels as prescribed. I was even trying to relax – by far the hardest thing for me – through weekly acupuncture sessions. My husband continued to be gently supportive of me and our situation, as he had been all the way through this journey.

The cycle went as well as it could, and they transferred two blastocytes at day five. Scan photos in our hands, we went home to wait and to hope. However, by the morning of the two-week blood test to see if I was pregnant, I already had an idea that it hadn't worked. I'd been taking home tests daily for the last week and they had all been negative. The nurse checked my contact details and said they would ring me in the evening with the results.

Expecting bad news, yet in denial that it was coming, I didn't cancel my evening clinic and so I saw my patients as usual. My only allowance was to leave a gap between appointments at the approximate time I would be expecting the nurse's call. When the phone rang with an unknown number, I walked quickly out of my consultation room so I wouldn't be disturbed, and down the corridor to the counselling room. This was a less clinical space softened by cushions, bright chiffon scarves draped over the backs of comfy chairs, and abstract paintings hung on the walls.

I answered the call.

'We're very sorry,' said the nurse in sympathetic tones, 'but the pregnancy test is negative. The cycle was unsuccessful.'

I thanked them for calling me, took a deep breath and rang my husband to let him know the bad news. I sat in the counselling room alone for several minutes, pulling myself together before going back to finish my clinic.

I don't know if my patients noticed anything different about me that evening. I doubt they could have guessed that I had just been given the news that meant that I would never become a biological mother. I swallowed my sadness down, kept calm and carried on until I went home.

I can only imagine how different things might have been if I had given myself the time and the space to properly absorb the news. To let myself be comforted when I got it. To start the grieving process from a kinder place.

This set the tone for my approach to grieving going forwards.

After our last treatment ended, I searched the internet to find out how other women had coped with infertility. I read blogs from women in similar situations and learnt that this coping is in itself a form of mourning. I understood that for me to move on, I needed to do grief work.

Grief work is described as the 'psychological process of coping with a significant loss' and was first conceptualised in 1944 by the psychiatrist and researcher Erich Lindemann in the *American Journal of Psychiatry*. He theorised that, for people to progress through grief to a place of healing, they had to actively do grief work. The type of work and the time taken for it varies for different people.

As infertility involves losses that may be invisible to others, much of this grief work is done in silence and isolation, unlike grieving the death of a loved one, which is more easily validated and supported by society. People may also be dealing with feelings of shame and self-blame, which can make talking about infertility with loved ones harder.

Work was something I always excelled in. As the child of Indian immigrants who came to the UK to work for the NHS, the value of hard work and achievement was instilled in me at an early age and reinforced by my own experiences of working in healthcare. I found comfort in it, believing that if I only worked hard enough, I could achieve anything I wanted. Being unable to bear a child shattered this illusion. However hard I worked, I couldn't control my body and change the outcome.

So I jumped in. From 2013, my grief work included attending courses, meeting brave and inspirational women coming to terms with childlessness, and having therapy. If people were offering gold stars for doing grief work, I would have got plenty.

But did I really do the work, or was I just ticking boxes? Course done – tick; peer support found – tick; therapy done – tick.

I remember during this time listening to a podcast episode

on which Jody Day, the pioneering founder of Gateway Women, the friendship network for those who are childless by circumstance, spoke about avoiding what she called 'Mother Teresa syndrome'. This is the idea that because you are childless you have to do something of enormous significance, as if to compensate.

I thought this was excellent advice, knowing myself well enough to understand that this was a trap I could easily fall into. However, I spent the next decade doing the exact opposite of following it. I threw myself into my job, which I loved, and volunteered for related charities and organisations in my spare time. Whilst this was incredibly rewarding and opened new and exciting opportunities, it also allowed me to pack up my sadness and put it away. I hid it from others and even myself, until it became a tiny part of me, as hard to see as those embryos in the scan photos.

At a party, an older relative told me: 'You really should get on and start thinking about having a baby. You're running out of time.' The night was ending, and he was drunk on beer, whisky, and the knowledge that he always knew best.

As he doled out this helpful advice, his wife gave him a sharp word and elbow in the ribs. I mumbled something to show he had been heard and walked off seething. I raged at my husband that I couldn't believe the thoughtlessness of the remark or the casualness with which it had been thrown at us. I wished I'd had the confidence to tell him that we had tried, but sadly it didn't work out for us. But shame held me back.

At this point, it was 2018 and we were more than five years on from our last IVF cycle. I thought we had been fairly open in telling our extended family that we had completed treatment and were coming to terms with being childless. My parents, and my sister in particular, had been helpful at spreading the word to relatives we didn't know well, or where there was a language barrier, so that we didn't have to.

But perhaps it wasn't entirely that relative's fault. If I had been less discreet about my pain and less anxious to show people I had moved on, he may have known not to make the remark. This is not to excuse him, but had I made too little of my sadness?

I now understand that if I couldn't see my sadness, or let it exist without hiding it away, was it any wonder that others couldn't see it? And by dismissing it, was I also dismissing and hiding my resilience?

As part of my grief work, I was advised to write about my fertility journey in the third person, as someone observing from a distance. I read it again for the first time in many years in preparation for writing this piece, and was struck by just how much had been thrown at us, and how we had coped. I've always had a niggling thought, 'Did we *do enough*?' and reading my account reassured me that yes, we did more than we ever expected to, but had bad luck. It wasn't our fault. Some things are not meant to be. Parenting can happen in other ways.

I feel grateful for this strange and unsettling year for giving me the head space to allow these insights, more of which are probably to come. I see my sadness now: it will always be here, ebbing and flowing at different times in my life, but I hope to embrace it and make friends with it. By acknowledging its existence, I will allow other people to do the same. I will let them know that I desperately wanted to be a mum, but it didn't work out for me. I will let them see both my vulnerability and my strength. I will truly be seen.

It's time for a kinder, gentler existence that includes mothering myself. Not being a strict mum, punitive when I don't meet my high expectations, but a supportive one who offers myself hugs and home-cooked food. I will understand that I have boundaries and limitations, so I can let myself rest and recover, and allow other people to look after me. And so, this essay is part of my grief work. Writing it has felt therapeutic, although I can't help wondering if it's also been something else to achieve – another tick box. I know it's not going to be easy to change the habits of a lifetime.

As I type this, I have some niggling pain in the left lower side of my abdomen. It's probably due to my endometriosis. I should close the laptop and take some painkillers, but I probably won't. Learning to be kind to myself is going be hard work – but I'm good at that. I am a work in progress.

*Rageshri Dhairyawan is a writer, sexual health and HIV doctor, and researcher. Her debut non-fiction book on how people go unheard in healthcare, and how this can be addressed, is due to be published in 2024.*

# Notes From Here

*Kat Brown*

*I* *have kept a diary on my phone for twelve years, largely because I lose everything else.*

## 6 April 2017

On the way to a family lunch, I snapped at H and dissolved into tears because I realised that I wasn't cross, I had PMT. Almost two years of solidly being aware of my body and feeling heartily sick of it. Guilt, guilt, shame, shame.

I had bought a large box of ovulation sticks from Clearblue, whose bloody YouTube advert had been stalking me all year with its nursery-rhyme refrain, '*Twinkle, twinkle YOU'RE PROBABLY BARREN.*' I weed on the sticks, got the flashing smiley face, and later the static smiley face. This time, maybe? No, my period came.

The next month I got eleven days of flashing smiles. It was like being haunted by the Joker. *Where is my ovulation? I deeply object to having to be this obsessed with my own eggs. It is difficult to take an interest in ones you cannot poach, scramble, or buy from Waitrose.* The smiley face never settled into certainty. I looked at one of my many apps and figured it must have happened, or the sticks were lying, or they'd just kept going because I'd done it wrong. Either way, my period was due in two weeks.

Except this time, it didn't come. One day passed, then two. Indoctrinated by Clearblue, I went to Boots to get an early detection test and went back to work dreading being pregnant. Terrible mother. End of my career. Child will probably hate me. What if I can't get it to eat anything?

*Not pregnant.*

What? Fuck off, I must be pregnant. I always came on when my app predicted it. I looked at the packet and realised I'd done the test wrong. For crying out loud. Another four hours 'til I could take it again.

I spent the rest of the day feeling cross and tried again. *Not pregnant.* I checked the internet and found lots of people saying they'd had false negatives for days afterwards, and then got it 'right'.

I was getting little prickly cramps, but still no period. The internet told me it was probably the egg planting itself in my womb. 'Nobody told me this would hurt,' I bleated to myself, ignoring the whole bit about childbirth, morning sickness, back pain and other thrills. The prickles continued, and no period. Four days late. Five. Six, seven. I must be pregnant.

I had a hen do on day nine and resolved not to drink. On day ten, I had a glass of prosecco at a friend's book launch.

On day eleven, I took the pregnancy test again. *Not pregnant.* My period rocked up shortly after.

At the same time as I started thinking, *This isn't fair*, parallel thoughts ran in. *It could have been so much worse. You didn't have a miscarriage. You could have lost a baby late term, or it been ectopic.* And yet, there it was, this tiny moment of nothing.

I cried so hard that I was an hour and a half late for work. I had lost . . . nothing. There was no reason to feel sad. And yet I cried, and cried, and cried, not at my failure this time, but for something that had never really existed – but, for the shortest time, just might have done.

## *14 April 2018*

My list of baby names is now covered in strike-throughs where people have laid claim by very rudely having a baby before me. I've started to respond to this in the same way as I do when I'm not immediately good at something: *If babies don't want me, then maybe I don't want babies!* If I see one grizzling, or one I just randomly take against, or who has an annoying parent, I go, 'Well, thank Christ I haven't got one of those.' But then I see my niece, or a friend's twins, and even if they are screaming, my heart tells me quite firmly that this is the most beautiful, wonderful baby on the planet and yes, wouldn't it be nice to have one too?

Enough babies have been born now that I feel like a wizened old man of the hills. Some days, I think, *Well, maybe this isn't meant for us after all.* And then I see H sitting with his nephew like two comfortable jigsaw pieces, and go, *No. We haven't even got started yet. Let's start soon.*

## *20 March 2019*

There is a café on the ground floor of our spotless new fertility centre. I ask the lady if she's got any decaf, and she smiles as if to say, 'Darling, this is the one place that's an absolute certainty.'

There's a little bunny doll in a ballet dress perched on the till, and I feel that familiar self-protective distancing I get when hospitals try to put me and the possibility of children in the same place. *Brace, brace! Prepare for the gentle crush of failure and the continued self-questioning about whether you actually want them anyway.*

I look at the food on offer and decide primly not to have any, having had three biscuits and then a load of cake at a lunchtime seminar. The thumping in my chest has calmed somewhat and I just feel very tired, accompanied by the roar of sugar.

Memories fly in like a dream sequence: the 'Effort Street' road sign outside our first hospital; the company delivering my IVF meds being called Stork, of all things, and every time I've ever seen an exhausted pregnant person and thought, *We-ell, it's your fault really, you're not ill – you chose this.*

I note blearily that, once again, it's usually women who have to deal with 'this'. We have to defend ourselves and our right to equality, equity and feminism. We have to grow the sprogs, going through the physical and mental misery of pre-paring over and over again for something that can, for whatever unexplained reason, simply not happen. I was so furious when I went to see the fertility counsellor. THIS IS TOO MUCH IN 2019.

More scans. When I was little, I had an ultrasound. I remember the cool feeling of gel on my tummy as the wand moved around, seeing what was inside. I never thought it was a baby or what mummies had, and I never have. I am having so many scans at this new, shiny, polished building with its certificate frames hanging empty that it gives me flashbacks to university open days. This could be yours! If you are clever, sexy, witty, wanted enough, you too could stride around as a member of our magnificent institution. But until then, please drink the free coffee, admire our glass tables, and go through the rigmarole of having scans while not being knocked up. This is just your open day. You aren't one of us.

*[22 March 2019, first cycle of IVF; Nine eggs collected, none mature enough to fertilise.]*

*26 March 2019*

From therapy:

- Only share something if it's healed
- Keep a temple in your heart
- Don't let trying stop you living
- Think, *Good for you and the same for me*

Infertility is like knocking at the door of a huge house you've been looking forward to visiting for ages, only to find out that nobody is waiting for you. It's incredibly lonely – waves of loneliness of the sort I recognise from depression. A helpless, high, hysterical loneliness, like being trapped under the ice away from the world.

*7 May 2019*

Me: 'It was so sad and hard.'
   H: 'Why? The hormones?'
   'The new baby in my head. I am grieving for the baby I

will not have. I am grieving for her. I had planned out her announcement in *The Times*. ('Thanks be to God and the NHS.') What would she have loved, this little daughter of ours? Would she be as capricious as her namesake? Would she have minded being named after a Jilly Cooper character? And our son – I had so hoped for three or four children, building a crowd. And now we may not even have one.'

'There are 14 million different timelines, and we don't know which one we are in.'

'I should never have taken you to see that bloody film.'

'What?'

'You just *Endgame*'d me.'

'Oh. Yes! But no – we *are* in a little bit of infinity. But I know that I would much rather be in a timeline with you, and no baby, than not to have you at all.'

## 12 May 2019

Why do I want to become a mother? I didn't, not in the beginning. Every month my period came became a sigh of relief: another month to ride, to drink, to carouse, to have an adventure rather than having my wings clipped.

The streets seemed to be full of toddlers whingeing and parents with lines developing down the sides of their mouths to match the ones in their foreheads. Adorable babies needing tons of equipment to be transported anywhere. Youth groups and family centres closing down. No sense of flexibility or possibility, just sacrificing your own life to make someone else's. And what had I achieved in my own? It wasn't exactly brimming over with worth.

A few months after we married, I came off the pill. I was

weeks into a new job when, to my horror, my period was late. *What will my boss think? She's literally just hired me, and now I'm pregnant; how disgustingly irresponsible.*

I trooped along to the Boots at Piccadilly Circus and bought a test, taking it to the till defiantly – nobody should hide it – but in the manner of an unexploded bomb. I wasn't pregnant. The relief was staggering! When I got pregnant, I thought, my worth would disappear. I have seen the campaigns, the work being done by 'Pregnant Not Screwed', and my career so far consisted of titles closing down, departments fired, and me cannonballing from job to job with sporadic periods of 'freelancing' and a couple of months on the dole aged twenty-five, where the helpful man at Peckham Job Centre suggested that I apply to be diplomatic editor of the *Telegraph* as it was 'in the same field'.

Every time a celebrity had a baby, I checked her age. If she was older than me, I breathed in relief. There was still time. I wouldn't inconvenience anyone, not yet.

[*13 May 2019, second cycle of IVF. Twenty-two eggs collected; none mature enough to fertilise.*]

*14 May 2019*

I cannot concentrate. I feel like I'm in a bubble, floating above the pavement, where time doesn't really exist. I'm slipping in my freelance work: I pitch a book review and then cannot write it. I can't do anything unless I absolutely have to. I feel like a piece of toffee being stretched and never getting to breaking point, just longer and further away from where I need to be, isolated from my regular life.

The longer I wait, the more I hope. It sneaks into the dark like gold, calmly holding me with artificial promise, or like when the Blue Fairy's light keeps nearly turning Pinocchio into a boy, but he keeps resisting. For the first few days of my cycle, I am resolutely calm and logical. Then I let myself daydream. I imagine every moment of seeing that positive pregnancy test, of being able to do one of the elaborate presentations that I see online (which Harry would loathe and which I would secretly adore because it would mean acceptance).

Then I could say things all bright and relaxed, like, 'Isn't it wonderful? You were so right – as soon as we took that holiday, it just all fell into place!' 'I know! I just relaxed and my body must have . . .' (here I might trail off and throw my hands upwards with a goofy smile à la Drew Barrymore) or, to that bitch at the hospital, 'You were right! Stress *is* bad for my womb! Thank God I gave up caffeine, and alcohol, and went to live in an induced coma until suddenly I woke up pregnant.'

I imagined I would *win* and that this time I would be different in how I reacted to winning. On the rare occasions that I have won anything, be it a pub quiz or an award, I have felt my world starting to cave in, as though a terrible mistake has been made. Nothing prepares you for the feeling when you lose. It's the sadness. You feel sad at films or about someone dying, but the sadness – the grief – my God. Everything solidifies to the finest, thinnest point. You want nothing so much as to disappear, but now everything revolves around this devastating polarity, and there is no way to escape it.

'Do you have anything you want to ask me?' says the embryologist at the other end of the phone, gently (and what a horrible job this must be when all you want to do is to help people be happy).

'I know the nurses need to call every day to check up, but I found that really difficult last time. Would you mind asking them not to? And if I experience any symptoms, I will call in?'

'Yes, of course. If you need to talk to me, you can call. Is there anyone with you?'

I wake up for a minute to the cooling Turkish eggs beside my copies of *Country Life* and *Slimming World*. With almost ridiculous timing, Bob Marley is on the radio, singing that everything's gonna be alright.

'My husband is in a meeting. He will be back later.'

'OK, Katherine. Please call me if you need to talk.'

I hang up and realise that I am sitting in a rainstorm of my own making. I ring Harry, but he doesn't pick up, of course. I need to message people now. I need to ask Iso to update the Jilly book club for me. I don't want to go back to any groups for a while. I message my friends and reply to my mum's WhatsApp.

Harry calls. 'I'm so sorry. It didn't work again.'

I pay the bill, leave the café, and try to think of people I can call. If I do tasks, I can fix things. Doing equals mending. Mum hasn't replied yet; she only checks her phone about once a day, so I call her. I can hear she has read it.

'It's a complete bugger for you, and you've been such a brave girl. You will get there, and you will look back and say, "Oh that's the route we came! How strange," but you will get there.'

I don't have anything useful to do or say now. I can only creak. 'I just want to be a mummy.'

### 10 July 2019

Things that make me happy:

- Eating at Hood
- Doing a completable task like buying something I need
- Dressing up for an appointment
- Feeling in the middle of my own life
- Being happy for people's pleasures and successes
- External validation: an email, a commission, a nice message, Instagram likes, Twitter replies
- Going home to Harry
- Waking up with Harry and Ambridge
- Clean sheets
- Everything being neat in its right place

### 11 November 2019

I am violently angry. I feel as restless as a tiger, only instead of glamorous, I feel like a giant suet pudding of rage. I am angry, I am resentful, I am every negative emotion in the *Sesame Street* canon, and I am ugly, ugly, ugly in how very real and impolite my emotions are. How DARE this be happening? Our happiness seems perched on the end of a needle, the happiness we are so lucky to have.

I feel tension unwinding behind my tongue, almost pleasurable. Every muscle and bone in my body finally has a purpose: to express my absolute fury at this untenable situation. For this moment, I am part of this rage; I am not carefully moderating it, as I do with my therapist when I say something upsets me and automatically qualify it with, 'Of course, other people have it far worse, I'm very lucky; I have my health/home/husband/working limbs/I'm not a Dickensian orphan stuck up a chimney.'

If someone has something nice, I don't have to do what I have trained my brain to automatically do: to carefully express the genuine pleasure I feel without it being stung to death by the scorpion of my rage and resentment of 'How fucking dare you, when it should have been me.' I don't have to make the beast beautiful, don't have to make our infertility palatable, don't have to worry about worrying our families or causing anyone upset. For now it is just me in this fire, and I am so angry I vibrate.

I am so bored of being reasonable, of being recovered, of being 'over it'. I am not over it. The choice has been taken away from us, and the only way we stand a chance of fulfilling this dream is by forcing ourselves into expensive, drug-fuelled laboratories.

This rage is primal, and I realise why we use that word: it's because there is nothing polite about it, nothing civilised. It is a drunken, furious soup of emotion, picked out in colours that weave into a shield that keeps you alive while isolating yourself from others. And then, just as the anger reaches its beautiful height, taking me away from everything traumatic and frustrating and just plain fucking awful, then come the tears, and devastation comes towards me until it is overcome by the gravity of misery and self-hatred and judgement, and smothers me in a drowning viscous liquid of pure miserable terror.

The people who understand are picked out like gold nuggets in mud, smiling at me: 'You are perfect. This situation is happening to you, and you are responding in the only way you can. The decision has been taken away from you. You are doing your best, and I understand.'

When I hear those words, the roaring of those feelings recedes until I am left on the shore of my emotions, alone and small, like a very lost stick figure who hasn't yet been coloured in and who desperately needs to know that somehow everything is going to be alright – but nobody can tell me that.

*10 December 2019*

When Genevieve sleeps, she clutches her tail to her like a teddy bear. She is so pretty and haughty for something the size of a medium box of tissues. Ambridge has taken up furious residence on my pillow.

I don't even know if I want children anymore. Maybe it's just my biological clock shouting, 'DON'T BE LEFT OUT.'

*20 Feb 2020*

I thought I had decades mapped out through raising a family – my family. A new course for us and these new people we didn't know. What is my purpose now?

From therapy: Embrace the darkness as a canopy. 'The darkness is beautiful, for how else can we shine?'

*7 April 2020*

David Kessler on Brené Brown's podcast.

- <u>The worst loss is always yours</u>
- Grief must be witnessed
- Vulnerability is love
- Count to three and step forward

## 10 August 2020

From therapy: suffering = pain x resistance

If those pain points weren't there, what would you be doing with your life?

If you couldn't fail, what would you do?

## 2 September 2021

From therapy:

- Depression
- BED*
- IVF
- Childlessness after infertility
- Problem drinking
- ADHD

If one of these were gone, the rest would feel more manageable.

I need to talk about it because I grew up believing in stereotypes. Life is complex, layered and full of joy, just as it has really annoying medical problems. People who have fun also go through this!

* Binge eating disorder

*6 April 2022*

From therapy: talk to Harry and tell close friends I'm depressed again. Acknowledge the depression. Start singing again.

Get serotonin from small wins of writing. Make time to enjoy horse riding, the job, seeing friends and a weighted blanket.

I have been prescribed a nap every day.

*25 April 2022*

What does change look like?

- Acceptance
- Not focusing on the bad
- Not pinning all my hopes on fixes
- Steady, consistency
- Progress
- Mastering mindfulness and meditation
- Mastering sitting with distress
- Acknowledging thoughts and then letting them get on with it

*30 November 2022*

Through the café's fairy-light-lined window, I saw a little boy pointing out each star and holly wreath to his mother. He was giggling, and in his joy he looked up at me and waved, that little old-fashioned crooked wave that all children do, like the Queen Mother, before they've entirely worked out how to use their hands.

I waved back impulsively, and he laughed. His mother laughed too and snatched him up in her arms and kissed him, whispering something to him in the eternal magic words of love. They got into a taxi that had been silhouetted in the darkness and stepped forward to reveal itself before enveloping them behind its doors and driving off.

# Imogen and Delilah

*Natalie Sutherland*

M y miscarriage almost ended my life, but it also changed my life in ways I never expected. That's not to say, for one second, that I'm glad I miscarried, because that would be, frankly, idiotic. But traumatic experiences have a way of melding themselves into your being and setting you on a path that, without that experience, you would never have found.

I lost my second baby at seven weeks but did not find out until my twelve-week scan. I had had a 'missed miscarriage', which is where the baby dies silently but the body continues to feel pregnant. A somewhat cruel and sadistic joke.

I had bled in my seventh week and visited the Early Pregnancy Unit twice to get help, only to be told there was nothing they could do, and I just needed to 'keep an eye on it'. I desperately clung on to the pregnancy feelings, which I still had, hoping that the bleeding was normal, as they'd said it could be, and nothing more serious.

I continued to 'feel pregnant' and this was the first time that I had felt any of those classic pregnancy symptoms. With my first pregnancy I had none of them. This time, however, I had morning sickness and a lust for red meat and jelly sweets. I weirdly enjoyed this physical manifestation of early pregnancy and used these feelings as a beacon of hope after that first bleeding. If I was feeling sick and having food cravings, I had to still be pregnant, right?

But what I wasn't admitting to myself was the feeling that something was gone. My breasts didn't hurt anymore. I felt alone. No longer feeling that 'togetherness' I had felt in my first pregnancy, just me and Delilah. But I ignored it, praying that everything was fine. The bleeding had stopped, and I wasn't in any pain, so everything had to be fine.

Lying on the bed, waiting for the scan to come up, I remembered the tears I had cried when I heard Delilah's heartbeat for the first time, the wonderful happy tears of a woman who was now a mum. When the sonographer asked if I was sure that I was twelve weeks pregnant, I thought, what a ridiculous question, couldn't she see from the screen that I was twelve weeks? When she said, 'I'm so sorry,' I heard a guttural, harrowing howl and was astonished that the sound was coming from me. It was loud. It was terrifying. I think I may have made a bit of a scene; the poor sonographer must have felt awful giving me that news and I'm usually mindful of others' feelings, but in that moment, I didn't care about her. What was she saying to me? Despite my earlier intuition (as it turned out), I could not comprehend that not only was I no longer pregnant, but I hadn't been pregnant for the last five weeks.

How could that be when I had been feeling pregnant? I was told that the sac had continued to grow, tricking my body. The baby likely died during that seventh week when I had the bleeding. That seventh-week bleed had occurred at a time when I had suffered a very stressful and shocking time at work, and I have no doubt that the guilt of that will stay with me forever.

Leaving the hospital no longer pregnant was indescribable. I felt anger I'd never felt before. I couldn't stop crying and Jon, my husband, didn't know how to console me; no one was consoling him whilst I wallowed in my grief. How I kept it together when we picked Delilah up from nursery I'll never know. But I hid my sadness from her, removing the books we had been reading together about becoming a big sister, hoping she wouldn't notice.

You may be wondering where the 'miscarriage almost ended my life' bit comes in. So far, so ordinary, as far as missed miscarriages go. But missed miscarriages are a bugger to sort out. First, we tried expectant management, where you simply wait for the body to 'expel' the foetus naturally. After a few weeks of nothing and a continued positive pregnancy test, we tried medical management. This was painful and pretty horrifying. Scans continued to reveal 'product', and so I had a procedure called an ERPC (evacuation of retained products of conception), my first ever experience of general anaesthetic.

Unfortunately, even after the ERPC I was still testing positive for pregnancy. It was now July and I had had my scan in April. I was told that my period would eventually come, and it would be fine. Nothing else for them to do.

By this time, I'd had enough. We moved from Cambridge to Wales so that I could be home. I wasn't coping and I needed to centre myself and try to stop spinning. Our move to Cambridge from London had been a disaster and I could no longer be the woman I had been: the breadwinner and go-getter. I was changed and I didn't recognise myself. My whole life had followed a carefully crafted linear plan and I was suddenly sensationally off course. I was adrift and drowning in grief. I needed a lifebuoy, and, in that moment, that was Wales and my family.

By August, as predicted, my period came. But this was odd. Sitting on the sofa I felt an internal gush and quickly sped up the stairs to the toilet. Blood was pissing out of me. It didn't stop for twenty minutes, and I had no idea what was going on. My only thought was that this must be the end, finally, of my miscarriage saga. I was finally getting the bleeding that I had associated with a miscarriage. Surely this was now the end.

September and October 2018 were months I will never forget. The volcanic bleeding was now happening regularly, and, like a volcano, I had no idea when it was going to erupt. I worried that I would be walking down the street and the bleeding would start, and once it started, there was no way to stop it other than to wait. Interesting side note: I had started driving lessons but had to stop them as I was worried that I would ruin the driving instructor's upholstery.

My first ambulance ride to the hospital occurred early one September morning when I woke in a pool of blood. Rushing to the toilet, I splattered blood on the walls and carpets. I later heard from my mum, who works with the paramedic's wife (it's a small town!), that he had thought they'd turned up to a massacre. This first hospital visit resulted in some pills and an appointment for a hysteroscopy.

Before I had a chance to have that appointment, I was back in hospital. I had woken up with the familiar wet feeling and ran to the toilet again. Jon was already at work, so it was just me and Delilah at home. As the blood poured, I started to feel hot and clammy and, even though I was sitting, I had that feeling in my head that you get when you stand up too quickly. Then everything went black.

I don't remember anything else after that until I heard Delilah calling 'Mummy' from her bed in a distressed state. I realised that I was on the floor, and I couldn't move. I called her to come to the bathroom and when she saw me, she said, 'Mummy, there's blood everywhere again,' totally unfazed. I asked her to get my phone so I could call my mum and 999, and she got me a pillow for my head, as I couldn't get up. Delilah sat with me and held my hand until my mum arrived. She was my little hero.

I was taken to hospital again and this time I stayed overnight, hooked up to IV drugs. I was also sporting a massive purple-and-yellow bruise on my cheek where I had smacked my face on the sink as I passed out and fell from the toilet.

I was given more drugs to stem the bleeding and a week later my hysteroscopy revealed no retained product (hate that term), and that my fibroids were outside the womb and therefore not causing the bleeding as they had assumed. Instead, I was diagnosed with dysfunctional uterine bleeding – they basically didn't know what was causing it. But to stop the bleeding I had three options: (1) get pregnant – this would stop the bleeding as it normally would during a pregnancy, and the hope was that my body would just sort itself out after the birth; (2) put in the Mirena coil – this would stop the bleeding but also stop us conceiving, as it's a contraceptive; or (3) hysterectomy – I was thirty-nine and this was simply not an option for me.

Whilst I was considering getting a second opinion, the decision was made for me, as a week later I was back in hospital, and this time it was serious.

An hour after going to bed on a Friday night, I was woken by the familiar wet feeling. Luckily for me, Jon was with me, but for him it was terrifying. He witnessed me fall into black-out, my eyes rolling into the back of my head and my whole body spasming. He thought he was watching me have a stroke and that I was about to die in front of him.

Paramedics were called but, in the hour it took them to arrive, things had calmed down. They took me to hospital anyway, out of caution. But when I arrived and they transferred me to the hospital bed, the volcano erupted again. This time it was clearly serious, as the people in the room multiplied and the instructions were frantic and direct. I was tipped upside down and given oxygen, as I was about to pass out again. I was given morphine, which made me feel sick and sent me a bit loopy. I was convinced I could hear music through the oxygen mask.

Hearing the words 'get gynae down here now!' shouted had me a little worried. Then came the forms to sign to give my permission for a hysterectomy, should that be needed to save my life. Left with no choice but to sign, I asked them to call my mum. I was scared and I didn't want to die. I didn't want to lose all chance of getting pregnant either. But the thought of leaving Delilah, then aged two, without a mum – with the chance that she would grow up not even remembering me – was too traumatic to contemplate. I prayed.

I was taken to theatre and the gynaecologist asked for my permission to put in the coil. I said yes. I was now resigned to my fate, and saving my life was more important than getting pregnant again. Many months later my mum told me that the doctor had warned her that they were fully expecting to give me a hysterectomy, as the doctor was not convinced that the coil would stop the bleeding.

On the way down to theatre I was handed a phone so that I could speak to Jon. I remember telling him that in the morning he should let Delilah watch the old *Pink Panther* cartoons, as we'd watched some together that day and when I'd put her to bed I'd told her we could watch some more.

When I came round from the operation, the anaesthetist immediately told me that I still had my womb, and I was so relieved. As I was in and out of sleep, hooked up to a blood transfusion, I saw my mum sat at the end of my bed reading her Kindle. She held my hand and her calmness in the face of the scariest night of my life allowed me to just let go and not worry anymore.

I spent the weekend in the hospital and received four pints of blood and gradually my colour returned. My mum told me that I was so yellow I looked worse than her own mother did on her deathbed. The doctors told me that when the coil had been fitted, it miraculously stopped the bleeding. A nurse, Wanda, sat me down and explained to me just how poorly I had been. They had had a crash team on standby, as they did not think I was going to make it. I had very nearly bled to death.

With the bleeding now under control, I could slowly try to get my strength back. The loss of blood had resulted in anaemia, and I spent the rest of 2018 and early 2019 trying to heal (which included breaking my wrist in Norway celebrating my fortieth birthday whilst watching the Northern Lights!).

Whilst the physical trauma had now ended, the emotional trauma was only just beginning. Stupidly, I didn't get any counselling after the miscarriage; the physical issues had been preoccupying my time somewhat. With the chance now to be still, I started to process. A friend of mine ran a creative writing and yoga retreat, which I joined. I'm not a writer or a yogi (especially with a now ruined right wrist), but it felt like a fun activity to do, just for me.

Unsurprisingly, the baby I lost was the only thing on my mind. Whilst we had lost the baby too early to learn the sex, I have always thought of her as a girl. During a yoga session where we all sat round in a circle and chanted 'om', I had the most transcendent experience. The vibrations through my body were electric. Tears flowed unstoppably from my closed eyes while I thought of her and my overflowing grief that I would never hold her in my arms or watch as she played and giggled with Delilah.

I wrote a letter to her. A letter which, after the weekend, I put away and couldn't bring myself to read again for a few years. As I say, I'm no writer, but this is what I wrote:

My baby girl. I miss you. I wish you were here. You are so loved. Delilah doesn't remember you, but she will. I'll tell her about you one day.

*I'm so sorry I couldn't keep you safe.*

*I'm empty without you.*

I want to try for another baby. Another body for you to come to me in. I want you back.

We had so many plans for us as a four. We're wonky without you. You are needed. You are loved.

I don't stop thinking about you. I see you in the face of other people's babies, the ones who made it here safely. I see you in Delilah when she plays, and I wish you were playing with her. She needs you. She wants to be your big sister.

I feel you here, in this space, holding me. I know you feel my love and one day we'll be together again.

Love Mummy xxx

You don't ever 'get over' a miscarriage. The grief is in your blood. She was our second child, Delilah's sister; she was supposed to make us a family of four. We had already started seeing our life with her in it and yet we have to continue without her forever.

As Delilah got older and started making friends at school, most of whom had siblings, the inevitable questions about when she could have a sister (never a brother!) started. In December 2019, fourteen months after my operation, I had the coil removed. Luckily, the bleeding did not come back and soon my periods started and all seemed to be fine.

But month after month we failed to get pregnant. I was over forty and so the chances were slim anyway, but I lived in hope (don't we all!). But it was not to be. I had secondary infertility. And then the pandemic hit and life as we knew it changed again. By this time, we had moved back to London and were both working, although now working from home.

In September 2021 we told Delilah about losing the baby. I needed her to know that we had tried for a sibling, but she had died, and Mummy hadn't been able to get pregnant again. Whilst she said she remembered me having to go to hospital and seeing all the bleeding, I'm not sure how much she really remembers.

Up to this point we had never named the baby. But Delilah named her Imogen, and I loved the name and loved that she now had one, from her sister. For a while, Imogen was all Delilah could talk about and I really began to wonder whether we'd done the right thing in telling her, as she would often get upset. Imogen was now included in Delilah's stories and in her drawings and whilst it was beautiful to see, it ripped my heart open again.

I started a new job as partner in a law firm, Burgess Mee, and after spending almost a year working from home, in the latter part of 2021 we were back in the office. In a partners' meeting in September, I shared my miscarriage experience. Prior to this, two colleagues had confided in me that they worried about their fertility and, remembering being a young solicitor trying for a family, I wanted to ensure that the culture in our firm was one in which our female solicitors knew they could share their family-building aspirations without fear of it impacting their careers. Whilst I knew the outcome that I wanted to achieve, I had no idea how to go about it.

My bosses suggested that I be the firm's fertility officer – it seemed so simple and so obvious! I was clearly trusted by the junior staff and had had my own fertility issues, which I was happy to share, and so I could bring that experience to the role. Importantly, it showed the staff that the partners considered this such an important issue that they had put in place a dedicated position.

I now channel my grief into helping others manage their own fertility issues, particularly as it relates to work. What started just as the desire to help our staff navigate fertility turned into a wider movement when I teamed up with Somaya Ouazzani to hold a panel event called 'In/Fertility in the City' in December 2021. Six senior female lawyers and coaches shared their individual fertility stories with a packed audience, who were visibly moved. I also shared my own miscarriage and near-death experience and told them about the fertility officer role, hoping that members of the audience would go back to their own firms and implement the idea there.

However, I was a bit shocked when the national media

picked up on the newly formed role and the whole thing took on a life of its own. Articles appeared in the *Mail on Sunday*, *The Times*, the *Sun* and the *Telegraph*. I was named 'the UK's first fertility officer' and overnight I had to find my voice when I appeared on *Woman's Hour*, interviewed by the fertility warrior herself, Emma Barnett. I say I had to find my voice because prior to this I was quiet and terrified of drawing attention to myself. I was worried about what people would think about what I had to say, and worried about saying the wrong thing and being ridiculed. But since experiencing my own traumatic fertility story and starting to advise clients in relation to fertility and surrogacy law, and now being a partner in a law firm which embraced my trauma and gave me an outlet to help others, I believe I have truly found my calling.

The fertility officer role has very quickly been needed in my firm, where I have helped colleagues who have experienced miscarriage and ectopic pregnancy and undergone fertility preservation through egg freezing. I am told by them that without this role and the visibility and safety that it engenders, they would have experienced these issues alongside their work in a very different way.

'In/Fertility in the City' has also picked up pace. We had our second event in July 2022, doubling our numbers from the first event and attracting more and more law firms, chambers, HR departments and, crucially, men to the conversation, and we also now host a podcast of the same name.

By sharing my story and the reasons why the fertility officer role is so important, I have gained amazing opportunities, such as assisting Nickie Aiken MP with her Fertility Treatment (Employment Rights) Private Member's Bill, which aims to change employment law so that everyone has the statutory right to paid time off for fertility treatment and employees don't have to rely on their employers putting policies in place. Helping to change the law will be such an incredible achievement.

Looking back on the traumatic year that was 2018 and comparing that version of me with this version, I am so proud of the journey I have been on and the person I have become. I will always wonder what my life would look like if Imogen were here. I still burst into tears at the scale of the loss. I still feel guilty about not being able to give Delilah a sibling and ache for what she is missing: not only siblings, but nieces and nephews in the future. I hope she reads this when she is older and understands that we tried.

I have never truly been as open as I have while sharing my grief. Having and losing Imogen has given me a voice. It has become my strength. A piece of my heart will always be missing, but I am so happy that speaking of her and sharing my story is creating positive change for others, leaving a legacy to be proud of.

*Natalie Sutherland qualified as a solicitor in 2006 and is a partner at Burgess Mee, where she heads the firm's Modern Families Department. In 2021, she became the first fertility officer in the UK and co-founded* In/Fertility in the City, *a podcast and live events series aimed at creating a culture shift in workplaces for supporting staff going through fertility treatment.*

# Hard Glad

*Stella Duffy*

I talk about this stuff. I've talked about this stuff for decades. But sometimes people don't want to listen. Sometimes we don't want to listen to ourselves.

These are some of the things I talk about.

March 2000. My thirty-seventh birthday. For the past six months, with the woman who has already been my partner for ten years, the woman who is now my wife, we have been talking with our dear friends about becoming parents. He will be our babyfather and she the fairy godmother. We have made plans, made our choices, talked it through and imagined any number of future scenarios. Working with a hospital fertility department to get our best chances possible, we have had counselling together to be sure this is what we each truly want. They didn't ask the heterosexual couples to have counselling first. We were good to go: all three of us – me, my now wife, our babyfather – had each been ticked off as fertile and sane enough; we had gained the fertility unit's stamp of approval. Then, in mid-January, just as we were about to begin trying, I woke up one Friday morning with a three-centimetre tumour in my right breast. Because I was young,

246

because breast cancer was not in my family (it is often not in families), the tumour took six weeks to diagnose, growing in that time, and finally it was confirmed, yes, I had breast cancer. Before surgery I was told I was not allowed to have my now-wife's name on the form; she was not my legal next of kin. I had to name a sibling instead. After surgery, on my thirty-seventh birthday, we went to speak to the oncologist to find out what next. Google is not a good friend to cancer patients, but I was already aware that the size of the tumour made it highly likely that chemotherapy and radiotherapy would be recommended, and that the chemotherapy I would be offered stood a high chance of sending me into early menopause, making me infertile.

The oncologist did indeed recommend chemotherapy and then looked a little shocked when I asked about my chances of keeping my fertility. It had not occurred to him that a lesbian woman might want children. After all, my now-wife, then partner, was not allowed to be listed on my intake form. To their credit, once we had clarified our situation, the cancer and fertility departments were very helpful, but I do not believe a heterosexual couple would have had to point out, in their thirties, that yes, they were considering becoming parents.

Coming out every day is what happens to queer people all the time. It is exhausting and frustrating. Coming out in cancer and fertility treatment is much more so. Even our own childlessness community could do a great deal more to reach beyond its heteronormativity to include all of us.

That year, in this order, I had biopsies, diagnosis, surgery, egg retrieval from which five embryos were created and frozen, chemotherapy, radiotherapy. In all, it took almost ten months. My wife became pregnant during my radiotherapy and subsequently miscarried. She never became pregnant again. At that time, I was a writer and performer, freelance. There was no possibility of sick pay or compassionate leave; I worked throughout. The informative material given to me about chemotherapy talked of the impact of hair loss. It did not mention the impact of fertility loss. Hair grows back.

June 2003. I am sitting on my mum's settee in her little almshouse flat. She is to the left of me. She is dead. We think her heart stopped at some point in the night. There is a shopping list on the coffee table in front of her; I was coming over to take her shopping and then out for lunch. This morning I went to acupuncture. Somewhere in my uterus is the last of the five embryos made before chemotherapy. The others have all died inside me. I sit beside my mother and am longing to touch her dead body, frightened to touch her dead body in case death is contagious. In case this embryo dies too. It does.

No one behind me, no one ahead of me.

Genetic loneliness is not something we talk about much, but it is there every time we hear our friends and family speak about their children, their grandchildren. I have glorious relationships with my fifteen nieces and nephews and their thirty-one children. I know the diagonals in a family tree matter enormously. And still, we live in a culture where the up and down of the parent-child is the prime relationship. It wasn't always; we in the wealthy white West used to understand the extended family far better than we do now, but since capitalism really took off in the twentieth century, since the post-war invention of the nuclear family, this is how many of us live, in small blocks of humanity. For those of us without children, for those without partners, the primacy of the 'hard-working family' is a constant exclusion.

After cancer, after the embryo losses, I got better, I carried on. I carried on hard. I worked, I wrote, I performed, I directed, I co-founded a UK-wide charity. And then I got cancer again. This time, after a while, despite my best endeavours, I was not able to carry on. Losses are cumulative; they build up. It has only been in the past five years or so that I have been able to access and acknowledge the pain of the deeply traumatic egg retrieval. The procedure was rushed so it could be squashed between surgery and chemotherapy, and the pethidine failed to work adequately in my body, which was already deeply pained, barely recovered from cancer surgery. It is only very recently that I have allowed the awfulness of one dead embryo after another, the final death coinciding with the death of my mother, my orphaning. Now I can admit to myself how hard it has been to live with these losses, with the exclusions our culture forces upon me in my queerness, my infertility, the chronic pain I live with as a result of cancer treatments. All of which are connected to my being alive today. In cases of ill health, it is rare that a gain does not include loss.

Perhaps we might say that no one talks about cancer-induced infertility because it's so bloody hard to talk about. It has been hard to allow myself to deeply feel these experiences and the feelings they engender. Our culture assures us that anger, bitterness, rage, envy, jealousy, resentment are bad feelings, that we shouldn't feel them; it's better for us to move on, to let them go, to ride them out. But, like any grief, we cannot get *over* it; to allow the grief is to go *through* it. All of it, including the hard and dark feelings that our loved ones often prefer us not to have. Allowing my fury at the ease with which some people become parents, and their blithe ignorance of that ease, their assumption of it as a right, not a privilege, allowing my anger at that prevalent pronatal attitude has also allowed that anger to shift. Allowing my envy and jealousies has transformed them. Allowing bitterness and resentment – those feelings that women, in particular, are warned against, lest we become unlovable crones – has been so valuable. Pretending I didn't feel them didn't help, and while feeling them has been bloody hard, brutal, it has also loosened them, unmoored me from their grip. I don't believe this going-through is a one-time thing. Like any grief, I know it will come back, but I trust that the waves will be less forceful for the experiencing and allowing.

We don't talk about these things because often it's just too much. Heterosexual couples who have a glimmer of how it might be for LGBTQ+ people sometimes feel a touch of shame that their marriages, their relationships, are so easily welcomed, recognised, allowed. People without a cancer in their own body perhaps feel lucky and grateful that they have not had to make the choice of fertility or chemotherapy. People whose babies arrive through choice and desire, in good health and happiness, look at the compound losses of others and simply do not know what to say. It can be hard to know yourself fortunate in the simple good ease of never facing a life-threatening disease, not losing embryo after embryo. But it is just good luck, and those who have that good luck no more deserved it than I deserved my bad luck.

Sometimes people find it hard to talk about these things because the things that are simple for some – citing your partner as your next of kin, living without illness, getting pregnant and the pregnancy lasting – are impossible for others. Sometimes the very existence of our losses reminds others of the precarity that underscores all of life, all of our lives. And that makes us, the loss-carriers, scary.

Talking is hard because words pin down, they define, they set. And so much of what we feel in loss needs to move, to flow. Stuck in our grief we become lost. Shifting as the grief shifts, one day a gentle trickle, the next a roaring flood, we can learn to flow with it. It is rarely easy or simple, but allowing loss to move through us is the only way to let it be. It is an embodied experience and needs to be in and of the body. Embodiment is hard to word, easier to move, to dance, to touch.

Another reason it feels as if no one talks of these things is because what happened to me didn't happen to you. Not in the way it happened to me, not exactly. And what happened to you didn't happen to me. Not the same, not quite, maybe nowhere near. There is no one who gets how it is for me, for you, for any of the individual writers in all those books out there, for any one of the many readers of this book. In our losses we are each alone. And that is hard. Our loneliness can feel impossible, but we can choose to bear that loneliness together. We can be alongside each other. Your losses and your gains are not mine, and even so, I can be with you in yours and you can be with me in mine. In this way, we might begin to talk about these things, not to promise understanding, or to arrive at a place where we all get it, but because an openness to the differences is as useful as acknowledging the similarities. No one talks about these things because they belong to each of us utterly individually – in sharing them we can offer each other another possibility of belonging.

Writing this has been bittersweet, reminding me of what I

have been through. Some of this writing has been far more bitter than sweet. It hurts to talk of these things and to write them. Putting words to my own losses, getting them out there again for the scrutiny of others, is hard. I've been out for decades. Coming out every day, as is so common for all queer people, is hard work. Coming out about my cancers is hard work. Coming out about my infertility is hard work. It is also – they are all also – valuable, if not to others (I cannot presume that my being out is useful for others, that is up to them), then to me. It is useful to me to name my truths, however hard. Naming them allows them both to be and to change. No loss is ever set in stone. Our grieving morphs; there are high tides and far shallows. Grief changes, if we let it. Part of letting it is allowing it to exist. Part of letting it is speaking of it. If we want others to speak of these things, then we too need to speak of them for ourselves.

About two years ago, after another few long months of really tussling with the lifelong implications of my cancers and infertility despite – or perhaps because I was – coming up to sixty, I reached a new plateau. It is where I am now, and it feels good. I allowed myself to really look at the shame I feel about my own internalised pronatalism, the places where I too have bought into the story that I am not a proper woman, not a graduate woman, not a real woman, because I am not a mother. Instead of protecting myself against the pain as I have often tried to do, reasoning it away, exhausting myself in work or activism, I dived into my losses of not-mothering and – through that fierce and wrenching, painful tussle – came to a slightly easier resolution than I had had until now. Part of what allowed me to get to this place was choosing to allow my envy and resentment of the so many taken-for-granted parentings, including those in my own family, choosing to let those feelings be, instead of denying them or trying to understand them away. Bitterness and resentment and envy and jealousy are valid and real, and they have their place. Denying them does us no good at all, despite our culture's insistence that they're not good for us.

I was talking with my therapist about my own work now as a therapist, my lived understanding, my version, of some of the things some of my clients experience. He said (while acknowledging it was going to sound clumsy) that he was glad the embryos died in me, because it gave me where I am now; this loss and resolution, this knowing, this person I have become. And I agreed with him; I agree with him. I said, however, that I need the glad to be hard-glad, because it has been bloody hard-won and will, I'm sure, take more effort yet, next time it comes around. And it always comes around.

I think we do talk about this stuff – and we don't. We don't because it hurts us, and it hurts other people to listen to us. Sometimes we wish that other people had the same story so they could understand exactly what it's like, and none of us have exactly the same story, so we feel lonely. And that is why we want to talk about it, even when we don't want to talk about it, because sometimes sharing makes the lonely and hard a little easier to live.

So, we do talk about it, it's just that we're often not heard. Sometimes we need to have things in and of our own bodies to hear them from others. It's like death. We have always talked about death, loss, grief – every culture has its own way to do these things – but when it happens to us for the first time, it feels as if we have never heard these feelings said, these experiences told before – and that's because most of us don't want to listen to stories of transition or loss until we experience it ourselves.

We talk about these things, and we don't; we don't talk about these things, and we do.

Both things are true.

So here I am, just turned sixty. Over twenty years ago five embryos lived and died in my body, in me. The body in which I now live, my body, which is my vehicle for being in the world, was a site of life and death for five possibilities. My body is a graveyard. I am alive. Both things are true.

I am much more than a not-mother. I have had the great privilege of an inter-cultural relationship that has lasted over thirty years; our legal system even caught up with us finally and allowed us to marry. I am the youngest of seven siblings, an aunt and great-aunt. I have been an orphan for decades. I am a writer, a theatremaker, a creative mentor, a therapist. I have had cancer twice, and I have paid the cost of my survival, paid dear. I live with the disability and pain repercussions of my survival. And I love that I am alive. My losses remain part of who I am, and they no longer feel as if they are all of who I am. From this softer and quieter place, I am hard-glad to be where I am now. My hard-gladness was gained through letting the losses be just what they are, no less, but also, and eventually, not more than the fullness of me.

If you are reading this and wondering about your own hard, your own glad, the possibility of a hard-glad that works for your life, let your feelings guide you. Your anger and bitterness and fury and hurt and resentment and jealousy and loss and envy all have a place. All of your feelings matter: the well-behaved feelings are not more worthy than the hard ones. Nothing will make your loss go away; grief is simply grief. And we need to talk about this as well – that we can create lives of great value, fierce joy and deep possibility *anyway*. We need to talk about the pain *and* the possibility.

*Stella Duffy is an award-winning writer of seventeen novels, over seventy short stories and fourteen plays. She is also an existential psychotherapist working in private practice and for a low-cost community mental health service. Her doctoral research is in the embodied experience of postmenopause. Her website is: www.stelladuffy.blog*

# Resources

*Therapy and counselling*

British Association for Counselling and Psychotherapy: Its therapist directory allows you to search by specialism and city to find properly qualified support. (bacp.co.uk)

Petals: A free counselling service to support women, men and couples through all kinds of baby loss. (petalscharity.org)

*Free support phonelines*

Fertility Network: This wonderful line is operated by two former fertility nurses. Whatever you're feeling (or want to ask), Diane and Janet are here to help. (Diane, Mon/Wed/Fri, 0121 3235025; Janet, Tues/Thurs, 07816 086694. Both 10 a.m. to 4 p.m.)

The Samaritans: If you're feeling awful but thinking 'I'm making a fuss; someone else needs this more than me,' it's time to pick up the phone. Calls are free (116 123, www. samaritans.org)

Sands: A safe, confidential place for anyone affected by the
death of a baby, whether long ago or recently. (0808 164 3332,
10 a.m. to 3 p.m. Monday to Friday and 6 p.m. to 9 p.m.
Tuesday, Wednesday and Thursday evenings.)

*Further reading*

Jennie Agg, *Life, Almost*
Ayòbámi Adébáyò, *Stay With Me*
Dr Amy Blackstone, *Childfree By Choice: The Movement Rede-
fining Family and Creating a New Age of Independence*
Sharon Blackie, *Hagitude: Reimagining the Second Half of Life*
Candice Brathwaite, *I Am Not Your Baby Mother*
Jen Brister, *The Other Mother: a memoir for ALL parents (not
the smug ones)*
Julia Bueno, *The Brink of Being: Talking About Miscarriage*
Zoë Clark-Coates, *Saying Goodbye*
Jilly Cooper, *Polo*
Jody Day, *Living the Life Unexpected: How to find hope, mean-
ing and a fulfilling future without children*
Ben Fergusson, *Tales from the Fatherland: Two Dads, One
Adoption and the Meaning of Parenthood*
Emma Haslett and Gabriella Griffith, *Big Fat Negative: The
Essential Guide to Infertility, IVF, and the Trials of Trying for
a Baby*
Alexandra Heminsley, *Leap In: A Woman, Some Waves, and
the Will to Swim/Some Body to Love: A Family Story*
Jessica Hepburn, *The Pursuit of Motherhood/21 Miles*
Lucy Inglis, *Born: A History of Childbirth*
Lottie Jeffs and Stu Oakley, *The Queer Parent: Everything You
Need to Know From Gay to Ze*

Yvonne John, *Dreaming of a life unlived: Intimate stories and portraits of women without children*

Alice Jolly, *Dead Babies and Seaside Towns*

Georgina Lucas, *If Not For You*

Claire Lynch: *Small: On Motherhoods*

Hilary Mantel, *Giving Up The Ghost*

Sophie Martin, *The Infertile Midwife: In Search of Motherhood – A Memoir*

Meg Mason, *Sorrow and Bliss*

Dr Anita Mitra, *The Gynae Geek: Your no-nonsense guide to 'down there' healthcare*

Paul Morgan-Bentley, *The Equal Parent*

Dr Liz O'Riordan, *Under The Knife: The Rise and Fall of a Female Surgeon*

Philippa Perry, *The Book You Wish Your Parents Had Read (and Your Children Will Be Glad That You Did)*

AJ Silver, *Supporting Queer Birth: A Book for Birth Professionals and Parents*

Pippa Vosper, *Beyond Grief: Navigating the Journey of Pregnancy and Baby Loss*

Miranda Ward, *Adrift*

Rosie Wilby, *The Breakup Monologues: The Unexpected Joy of Heartbreak*


*Podcasts*

*Big Fat Negative*
*Everything Happens*
*Fertility Life Raft*
*Freezing Time*
*In/Fertility in the City*

*(Re)Defining Parenthood*
*Some Families*
*Unfertility*

*Online communities*

Black Mums Upfront (UK): Events, blogs and podcast from women who talk about all aspects of motherhood with a variety of guests. (blackmumsupfront.com)

Dope Black . . .: Support groups created by and for Black men, women, mums, dads, and queer people. (dopeblack.org)

Fertility Network: Support groups for Black women, South Asian women, LGBTQIA+ people, infertile men, male partners, childless people, under-25s, over-40s and single women – among others! (fertilitynetworkuk.org)

LGBT Mummies: A global channel offering live events and online support tailored to support LGBT+ women and people on the path to motherhood or parenthood. (lgbt-mummies.com)

Lighthouse Women: Previously known as Gateway Women, founded by Jody Day, this ID-checked online community for childless women has bespoke groups for all experiences. (lighthousewomen.org)

Paths to Parent*hub:* This community for people embarking on donor conception also offers specific support for LGBT+ people. (pathstoparenthub.com)

*Events*

Reignite Weekends (UK, Australia, USA, online): Practical events offering support and forward planning to childless women. (gateway-women.com/event-directory/)

Saying Goodbye Services (UK, France, USA, online): The Mariposa Trust's non-denominational services take place in beautiful buildings, giving people a chance to grieve a child they've lost. All services are explicitly open to everyone regardless of circumstance, including people who have not had the opportunity to conceive. (sayinggoodbye.org)

*Organisations*

Bliss: For parents of sick or premature babies. (bliss.org.uk)

Endometriosis UK: In-person and online support groups, events, information and support. (endometriosis-uk.org)

Five X More: Grassroots organisation empowering black people to make informed choices and advocate for themselves throughout their pregnancies and after childbirth. (fivexmore.co.uk)

Gingerbread: Working with the 2 million single-parent families in the UK. (gingerbread.org.uk)

Sands: The Stillbirth and Neonatal Death Society supports bereaved families with in-person and online meetings, and the Sands FC football teams for grieving male relatives. (sands.org)

Tommy's: For anyone affected by baby loss, stillbirth, miscarriage and neonatal death. (tommys.org)

TransUnite: Directory of in-person and online groups for trans people throughout the UK. (transunite.co.uk)

# Acknowledgements

*Kat Brown*

I described this as 'a support group in a book'. First of all, thank *you* for supporting me and for trusting that this endeavour would happen. I am so thrilled that you are a part of this and underlining the need to talk about what happens when 'family planning' doesn't work out that way. A huge thank you to everyone who wrote to me in public submissions – 'honour' is a hideously overused word, but to read your experiences shared so selflessly was just that.

Thank you to my parents, Jane and Richard, my brother Nick, and my favourite trio, Suzie, Florence and Annabel. Thank you to Nigel, Sarah, Cecily, Stuart, Archie, Jenny, Jack, Amy, Hannah, James, Deborah, Andrew, and all at LP – army of beloved niblings especially. To Stella Duffy, Nana-Adwoa Mbeutcha, Jody Day, Sophia Money-Coutts, Rageshri Dhairyawan, Gemma Stone, Noni Martins, Laura Barton, Alice Jolly, Seetal Savla, Miranda Ward, Yvonne John, Alice Rose, Donald Mbeutcha, Hilary Freeman, Quinn Clark, Tom Wateracre, Sarah Lewis, Emma Duval, Rosie Wilby and Natalie Sutherland. You have shared so beautifully and with such integrity. Thank you for being excellent (and prompt) contributors.

Thank you to my agent, Millie Hoskins, for not immediately sacking me when I cheerfully told her I was about to crowdfund £20,000 for a book for which I would be paid £0, and for being a steadfast cheerleader even when evidence/wisdom showed otherwise. To Katy Guest, Hayley Shepherd and Kate Quarry for sensitive, thoughtful (and blissfully thorough) edits – editing makes writing the best it can be, and it is a joy to have. Thanks also to DeAndra Lupu, Imogen Denny and Marissa Constantinou for further editing, and giving my husband cause to compare editing with the unfortunate turnover of drummers in Spinal Tap, and to all at Unbound for their beautiful work – Suze Azzopardi and Rina Gill, and Mark Ecob for a lovely cover without so much as a hint of my most loathed infertility trope, Woman Looking Forlornly Out To Sea.

To Pippa Vosper and Georgie Lucas, who I met through fangirling their invaluable books, for support, encouragement (and lunch), and to Helen O'Hara and Helen Zaltzman for their wonderful advice and reassurance. Thank you also to Rachel Dobson for Boggle; the Jilly Book Club for screaming joy; the Hamilton group for Eurovision and being appalling daily; N LYCN NC TCNTST NTS for the best quizzing; and Alice Hutton for making our identical cats go on a blind date over Zoom. I'm sorry Ambridge spurned Roland, but she is basically evil.

It's never ideal to have a hip replacement, still less to have a massive infection afterwards, which means your brain is candyfloss for three months. Thank you to the community nursing team at Gracefield Gardens for drugging me up every day, despite the efforts of an anxious golden retriever to be included. Thank you to Dr Carolyn Hemsley and her incredible OPAT team at Guy's Hospital, not least for going above and beyond to find me an antibiotic that made things a bit more normal. To Nicky and Simon Jones for their eternal excellence and access to supportive equipment, which I hope to return some time before 2036. To Annabel O'Connor, for quite literally picking me up when I was bleeding profusely into a towel and scraping me into the car to go 300 yards up the road to the GP – a legend is you, Acorn Productions. And Jonny Cook, without whom I would be but a panting potato on the floor.

This book's title is both accurate and ironic, given all the people who have gone before and who *have* spoken about this stuff, both publicly and in private. I am so privileged to have some of them writing here, alongside people discussing infertility publicly for the first time, and I hope this goes some way to helping others to speak about it, and to feel less alone, if but for a moment. Finally, to Fiona Lensvelt, who commissioned this book and held my hand even while delivering her own book (*Wild Card*, superb!) and also *a literal child*. This is for you, with love.

*Jody Day*
Thank you to Olafz, Gillian, Amanda, George, Caroline and Chloe for making me so very welcome in Ireland. To Laura Carroll for writing 'The Baby Matrix' and opening my eyes to pronatalism. And Mark, always, for Elly.

*Emma Duval*
Thank you to Kat Brown, your persistence and drive to see this book come together are truly inspiring, and to my

husband, for your support and encouragement each and every day.

### Yvonne John
I'd like to acknowledge my parents for moulding the creatively resilient queen that I have become and my partner, Cleve, for truly seeing me for who I am and loving me through my flaws.

### Alice Rose
Simon, always.

### Hilary Freeman
Thank you to the wonderful doctors, nurses and midwives in the Fetal Medicine Unit at UCH, who supported me through my pregnancy and Elodie's birth, and to the charity ARC, who helped me make the most difficult decision of my life. Love and thanks to Mickaël and Sidonie – for everything.

### Quinn Clark
In forty words I want to thank
All those who made this book:
The writers and the editors
And all those who'll have a look.

I've never been this open
And may never be again,
But I hope this vulnerability
Will soothe your restless brain.

*Seetal Savla*
For Neil, who encouraged me to find my voice and to keep using it to make a difference.

For Meghna, may we help you to discover yours and do what makes your soul sing.

*Miranda Ward*
Thank you to the healthcare professionals who've met my sadness with kindness. Carrie Bruce, whose wisdom and generosity has been a lifeline. The staff at the John Radcliffe Hospital maternity unit, who safely delivered my baby in a pandemic. Long live the NHS!

*Nana-Adwoa Mbeutcha*
It is only by God's grace that I have been able to share this experience so candidly – I pray it makes a positive impact on all those who need to hear it. Donald, I failed to see you before – I won't make that mistake again. Thank you for your vulnerability, thank you for your strength. Kiddos, thank you for reminding us of the beauty and sanctity of life for those born and those unborn. You've done your sister proud.

*Tom Wateracre*
I would like to thank Sarah Dean, Ian and Gill Davies, Terry and Pauline Dean, Simon and Catherine Hayes-Dean, Stef Ahlemann, Folakemi Akinbolade and C.

*Donald Mbeutcha*
To all the dads who have lost their angels and the dads who have created space for other dads to speak about their

loss – thank you. To my grandad and to my brothers, who have shaped me into the man that I have become – thank you. Of course thanks to Angela, who teaches me every day how to be a better father and man. And to God, the ultimate father of fathers – to Him always be the glory.

*Sarah Lewis*
Gratitude and thanks to Michael Kaufmann, who helped me reconnect with the light.

*Rageshri Dhairyawan*
Thank you to my family and friends for their love and support over the years. Thank you to Darren Chetty for always being there, for your love and for giving me the courage to write this story.

*Natalie Sutherland*
To my darling daughter, Delilah, you are the love of my life, and I am just in total awe of your awesomeness. To my husband Jon, my rock, I love you. And to Imogen, I love you and miss you every day. Kisses from Mummy.

*Stella Duffy*
I offer my thanks and deep gratitude to the NHS staff and services who have kept me alive long enough to tell this story.

I offer my thanks, deep gratitude, and love to Shelley Silas who is at the core of the life I am glad to live.

# Trigger Index

# Remembering Our Children

We remember with love the children who died, who couldn't stay, or who weren't conceived – and we keep them and their parents, friends and families close in our thoughts.

All the children we hoped for.

Araya and Leo Cutler, our little embryos. We will always love and miss you.

Ava Watts – who is loved to the moon and back.

Phoenix Benson

Busby babies

David (Didi) Dampney

Dorothy Rose Beverley Dring

Effie

Elizabeth Jane "Libby" King, Christopher Allen Eastman.

Eva and Emil, our beloved children in our hearts.

For H, always in my dreams x

For my baby, who I never got to meet. I wish you could have stayed.

For our would-have-been twins.

For the babies that didn't live and the people who grieve them.

For the four who didn't make it, and the precious one who did.

Max French

Rosemary and Lavender Freston-Hargrave

Sam Gough

Nicole Heaver

I'm sorry I couldn't have you.

In memory of all the babies of my friends and family who weren't able to stay with us but will always be remembered.

In memory of my elder sister, born sleeping 23rd May 1965. Known only as Baby Leake, now she can be named and her life marked: Jessica, you are not forgotten.

Isabella, Poppy and all the other baby names not used.

Chloe Lee

Little Dot

Emily Maud

My Seven Stars

My three children

My two babies, never met, 2012 and 2018. X

Ness

Nicholas John, aka Spike Cape Town 1986

Imogen Nicoll

Oakley, Westley, Hanley, and Lux Hamann

Our beautiful boys Francis & Gabriel Taylor. A moment in our arms, a lifetime in our hearts.

Our dearest Pumbaa. Forever our child and Alexander's elder sibling.

Our first son, Daniel Hibberd, big brother to Leo.

Our six precious babies in Heaven.

Eden Prevett

Remembering Clara with love.

Remembering my precious Timon, Pumbaa, Barney and Rupert – until we meet again.

Remembering our little fish, with all our love.

Richard Liam and Elizabeth Susanna – lost but not forgotten.

James Smith

Viola Testa

The three we never got the chance to meet – you are much missed.

Thomas Haynes – my always little brother.

To my three beautiful possibilities. I hope I get to meet you someday. xxx

Marcus Valette

Benedict John Peanut Yoxall

## Supporters:

Sophia Andeh

Fay Andrews-Hodgson

Lizzie Ayre

Sandra Baker

Daniel Bowden

Mike Brown

Bethany Buddery

Ruth Busby

Debbie Challis

Jade Concannon

A Cumming

Rochelle Cutler

Cortney Cynefin

Lesley Dampney

Natalie K Davis

Juno Dawson

DeafGirly

Isabelle Defaut-Juneja

Carrie-Ann Dring

Louise F

Manisha Ferdinand

Madelaine French

Linda Galloway

Ros Gough

Kate Gregory-Smith

Monica H.

Ellie Haworth
Jane & Matt Henaughan
Mel Spencer and Peter
  Hibberd
Anna and Nick Ireson
Dolly Jones
Sophie Jones
Alysia Kay
Jennifer King
Roxy L
Rosa Lamche
Heather Leake Date
Rebecca and Dafydd Lee
Katie Lee-Hall
Rachel Lewis
corey jo lloyd
Elaine Lomenzo
Sara R.T. Malhotra
  (GTD Survivor)
Clive and Naomi Matthews
Lizzie Bailey & Leah
  Matthews
Catherine Anne McCue
Sabine McEwan
Iona McLaren
Ben Mills
Sarah Murphy
Sophie Newbound
Emma O'Brien
Bree Oliver-Moss
Melanie Peake

Dr Annie Peppiatt
Francesca Perry
Nat Pinney
Sara Pont
Charles and Daisy
  Powell-Chandler
Yvonne Prevett
Marie Carlsen Ravnmark
Sue Reed
Kate Roberts
Gavin & Jen Roberts
Kim S
Natalie Mazhindu Sandock
Laura Schofield
Annabel Shepherd
Laura Shepperson-Smith
Alice Smith
Natalie Sutherland
Emma Tansey
Victoria Taylor
Sara and Liam Thacker
Kelly Tichy
Eleanor Turney
Andra Maria Valette
Zoë Veal
Katherine Wheatley
Jo Wheeler
Debbie White
Lucie, Merry and Willow
katy woodcock
Pippa Wright

Unbound is the world's first crowdfunding publisher, established in 2011.

We believe that wonderful things can happen when you clear a path for people who share a passion. That's why we've built a platform that brings together readers and authors to crowdfund books they believe in – and give fresh ideas that don't fit the traditional mould the chance they deserve.

This book is in your hands because readers made it possible. Everyone who pledged their support is listed below. Join them by visiting unbound.com and supporting a book today.

Chance A-R
Marion Acworth
Samantha Adam
Martha Adam-Bushell
Jennie Agg
Isobel Akenhead
Ruth Alexander
Kelly Allen
Aurelie Ambal
Frances Ambler

Bernice Ambrey
Rachael Anderson
Helen Anstee
Sharon Appleby
Charlotte Appleyard
Simon Arloff
Kristina Aschenbach
Ellen Austin
Rebecca Avery
Sarah Ayub

Michaela Azavedo
Cathryn B
E. B.
Claire Baker
Caitlin Baker
Katherine Baldwin
Jane Ball
Liz Barman
Becky Barnes
Tosh Barnes
Aimee Barnes-Austin
Duncan Barnett
Damian Barr
R.A. Barr
Tara Barry
Jill Barton
Jennifer Bartram
marisa Bate
Esther Beadle
Rachael Beale
Lexi Beam
Sheryl Beck
Katherine Beckett Suter
Katherine Bellenie
Tilly Berendt
Maria Berntsson
Adrian Berry
Diana Best
Hazel Bevan
Chris-Louise Bevell
Karen Beynon

Lori Bianco
Jessica Bifield
Sue Biggs
Julia Birch
Lisa Sara Bird
David Blackett
Marga Blankestijn
Nicola Bloor
Paula Bolton
Louise Boone
Alex Booth
Nina Börnecke
Amy Bottomley
Lesley Boughen
Anna Bowen
Helen Bowie
Heather Boyd-Savidge
Jen Boyle
Sarah Bradley
Meadbh Brannagh
daniela Brawley
Isabelle Bristow
Susannah Broadbridge
Ed Brody
Jo Bromilow
Gemma Brough
Mariko Brown
Nicholas Brown
Isabella Brown
Jane and Richard Brown
Beth Brumbaugh

Becky Brynolf
Daisy Buchanan
Nicki & Paul Burgess
Joey Burke
Anna Butcher
N Butcher
Katie Byrne
Sue Byrne
Christabel Cairns
Angie Caldwell
Ben Cameron
Hayley Campbell
Miana Campbell
Anne Campbell
Inês Campos Matos
Sarah Cantillon
Francesca Caracciolo
Orin Carlin
Katharine Carr
Ali Carroll
Holly Cartlidge
Karen Cartwright
Clementine Cecil
Laura Cervini
Leanne Chandler
Thalia Charles
Kate Chedciala
Carly Cheeseman
Will Chegwidden
Darren Chetty
Rageshri Chetty

Dushy Chetty
Jacqueline Christian
Sandy Christiansen
joanna christie
Rosie Clarke
Anna Clarke
Sarah Clement
Lara Clements
Brigid Coady
Rachel Cocker
Claire Cohen
Jamie Colaço
Teddy & Rafe Coleman
    Opperman
Jess Coles
Bea Colley
Lucy Collins
Kate Collins
Kathryn Collins
Mayumi Coloma
Chantelle & Ashley
    Connick
Emma-Marie Connolly
Selina Conroy
Sara Conway
Nick Cooper
Rachel Cooper
Henrietta Copeland
Poppy Corbett
Rachael Corn
Charlotte Cornell

Alex Costa
Luke Costello
Charlie Coulthard
Rebecca Cowley
Catherine Cox
Lizzie Craig
Caroline Crampton
Lynda Creber-Davies
stephanie creff
Elizabeth Cregg
Alexandra Crichton
Susannah Crichton-Stuart
Margaret Critz
Rachel Crowley
Julia Croyden
Lisa Cunningham
Fiona Curley
Jamie Dahlberg, MA, LMFT
Alison Dangerfield
Jon Dave
Lauren Davidson
Natasha Davie
Tom Davies
Ellie Davies
Eleanor Davies
Laura Davis
Lisa Dawson
Andy Day
Jody Day, Gateway Women
Ben de Pfeiffer-Key
Lizzy Dening

Lesli Desai
Sarah Deverill
Doyle Diane
Nancy Dickie
Matt Dixon
My-Hanh Doan
Rachel Dobson
Kristen Dolan
Rossa Dooley
Nina Douglas
Sarah Douglas
Rachel and Stuart Douglas
Abi Dowling
Susan Dowrie
Sian Dowson
Fonce Drake
Steven Draper
Sarah Draper-Gammon
Lynne Drew
Zandile Dube
Emma Dudley
Cliona Duffy
Katy Dunn
Annie Durham
Emma Duval
Hermione Eagle
Clare Eason
Ebona Eastmond-Henry
Gillian Eastwood
Sarah Ebner
Nicky Edmonds

Claire Edwards
Karen Edwards
Rachel Edwards
Sina Eißfeller
EK
Loulla-Mae
  Eleftheriou-Smith
Camilla Elphick
Miriam Elze
Laura Evans
Rhiannon Evans
Fi Evans
Harriet Evans
Rhiannon Evans
Carly Fabian
Emily Falconer
Rebecca Farrelly
FBG
Jessica Fellowes
Ninette Fernandes
Charlotte Fiander
Natasha Fielden
Gayle Findlay
Joyia Fitch
Clementine Fletcher
Nina Flitman
Sophie Flynn
Charlotte Forbes
Morag Forbes
Victoria Ford
Emilia Foster

Leonie Foster
Richard Foulkes
Oli and Hannah
  Franklin-Wallis
Melanie Frean
Agnes Frimston
Nell Frizzell
D Frost
Imogen Froy-Michel
Emma G
Ian G
Kirsty Gamble
Taylor Gamell
Kate Garchinsky
Cat Garruto
Laura Gault
Joanna Geary
Naomi Geidel
Celyse George-Gordon
Adele Geras
Rina Gill
Finola Glacken-Smith
Victoria Glass
Katie Glaze
Caroline Goldsmith
Laura Graham
Ali Gray
Jane Greaves
Araminta Greaves
Sallie Greenhalgh
Hugh Greenish

Elaine Gregersen
Catherine Gregory
Gabriella Griffith
Ray Griffiths
Nancy Groves
Hewete Haileselassie
Johanna Derry Hall
Ellie Hames
Cassie Hamilton
Lizzie Hampson
Amy Hamson
Katriona Hannon
Gill Harper
Sherryl Harris
Dan & Cat Harris
Georgie Harrison
Megan Harrison-Lund
Chippy Harrod
Horatia Harrod
Kayleigh Hartigan
Emma Haslett
Hannah Hastings
Peter Hawkins
Laura Haxton-Wilde
Paul Hayes
Beccy Heath
Sally Heiser
Katja Helenelund
Alexandra Heminsley
Melissa Hemsley
CSC Henderson

Cheryl Henderson
Hanna Hewins
Jennie Higgs
Mike Hills
Danielle Hines
Anna Hirst
Gabrielle L Hiscock
Suzanne Hodson
Kirsten Holt
Rachel Holt
Dieuwke Hooft Graafland
Kat Hopps
Anna Hornbostel
Brigitte House
Charlotte Hubback
Tanya Hubbard
JoJo Hudson
Joanne Hunter
Chloe Hunter
Alice Hutton
Helen Idle
Susie Imholt
June Indrefjord
Nicole Ingerson
Rebecca Jack
Rachael Jackson
Shelly Jackson
Jackie Jackson
Cecily Jenks
Elizabeth Jenner
Helen Jenner

Sophie Jennings
Anita Jensen
Jim & Di
Sophie Jobling
Yvonne John
Laura Johnson
Charlotte Johnson
Bryony Johnson-Newell
Alice Jolly
Jules Jones
Beth Jones
Zoë Jones
Eleanor Jones
Rachel Jones
R Jones
Paula Jones
Bianca Jones
Jessica Jordan
Laura Jostins-Dean
Julie Joy
Helen Judson
Vanessa K
Lauren Kaeding
Shona Kambarami
Melissa Karsenbarg
Daisy Kate
Andeep Kaur
Sarah Kaye
Sonal Keay
Sarah Kelleher
Katie Kennedy

Laura Kennedy
Al Kennedy
Deirdre Kennedy
Anna Kenyon
Lucie Kerley
Teri Kerr
Katie Khan
Malgorzata Kidd
Dan Kieran
Jane Kimberley
Rachael King
Will King
Annie Kirby
Vicky Klare
Sue Knox
Catherine Kodicek
Sandra Kolar
Helene Kreysa
Parimal Kumar
Eliza L
Carla Lafleur
Laura Lander
Laura Langan
Hannah Langford
Alice Langley
Charley James Lawrance
Chloe Le Breton
Cethan Leahy
Alex Lee
Alice Lee Holland
Lisa Lennkh

Max Lensvelt

Fiona Lensvelt

Joana Letra

Beth Lewis

Jackie Lidgard

Charlie Lindlar

Alex Lines

Samantha Lloyd

Helen Lock

Sara Lodge

Rebecca Logan

That Lot

Gemma Loughran

Jess Love

Elizabeth Lowson

Georgina Lucas

Kathryn Luke

Claire Luke

Natasha Lunn

Marit Elise Lyngstad

Anj M

Lisa Macario

Emily Macaulay

Eilidh Macpherson

Claudia Mahoney

Liane Maitland

Cesca Major

Kristine Mallett

Vicki Manning

Lauren Manson

Jessica Marchant

Sarah Markham

Sharon Marks

Laura Marmolejo

Linda Mason

Harriet Mason

Alexandra Matthews

Lizzie May

Katie Maynard

Kerrie McCabe

Katherine McCormick

Dani Mceneaney

Jo McGilway

Kate McGoey

Lucie McInerney

Gemma McIntyre

Deborah McIrvine

Carly McIver

Emma McKay

Esther Mckelvie

Faye McLoughlin

Vanisha McManus

Luke McManus

Krissy McNeill

Elizabeth Meager

Clare Elleray Mee

Amanda Mehta

Sarah Mercer

Hannah Michael

Laura Millar

Nick Miller

Kate Miller

Helen Milligan
Rachel Millington
John Mitchinson
Sophia Money-Coutts
Mim Monk
Claire Monkhouse
Emily Moore
Portia Morris
Frances Morton
Sheetal Morzaria
Hopeful Mother
Michelle Motherway
Helen Moulton
Abebech Moussouamy
Sofia Moutinho
Richard Moynihan
Alice Mpofu-Coles
Jo Mueller
Adrian Mules
Kat Munn
Kathryn Murphy
Beth Murray
Justin Myers
Rachel Myers-Girling
Karen Napier
Carlo Navato
Jonjo Neeves
Niamh Nestor
Ali Nicholl
Emma Nicholls
Catriona Noble

Claire Norman
Lucy North
Carol-Ann O'Connor
Kevin and Annabel
   O'Connor
Helen O'Hara
Lottie O'Conor
Ruth O'Loughlin
Kate Oldridge-Turner
Lizzy Oliver
Kate Olver
Mairead OMalley
Caryn Onions
Unn Inger Oreberg
Kylie Osborn
Jennifer Osborne
Anna Osbourne
Lizzie Ostrom
Susannah Otter
Jo Ouest
Naza P
Sophie Painter
Rebecca Palma
Liza Palmer
Anna Parke
Fiona E Parmanand
Claire Parsons
Karla Parsons
Danielle Parsons
Laura Pattison
Caroline Pearman-Gibbs

Abigail Pearson
Katy Pegg-Hargreaves
Rachel and Cora Marie
  Penny
Jenni Penrose
Cathryn Peppard
Josh Perry
Tiffany Philippou
Tom Phillips
Helen Pidd
Molly Pierce
Clare Pierce
Nev Pierce
Lisa Piercy
Kate Pleace
Margot Plews
Natasha Poliszczuk
Justin Pollard
Kiome Pope
Helen Pope
Anne Potter
Laura Potter
Nicole Powell
Marianne Power
Rachael Powers
Sonja Prakash
Beverley Presly
Laura Price
Rhiannon Pritchard
Alex Pruciak
Grace Rae

Jenny Raettig
Nicola Raimes
Natalie Reed
Jana Reetz
Lynne Reid
Angela Reith
Phoebe Reith
Catherine Renton
Amy Richardson
Robin Riley
Rebecca Rimmer
Lucy Riseborough
Rachel Roberts
Josi Robson
Rosie Ross
Sally Rowbury
Sophie Rubenstein
Charlotte Runcie
Megan Russell
Eve Russett
Emma Russo
Clare Ryan
Julia Sandiford
Rachael Saul
Jenna Saysell-Bailey
Rebecca Schiller
Holly Scott
Hilary Scott
Julia Searle
Catherine Seipp
Katy Seppi

Leanne Sermanni

Ruth Setz

Imogen Shaw

Marnie Shaw

Monique Shaw

Harriet Shearcroft

Angela Shepherd

Lucy Sheppard

Liz Sheppard

Nuala Sheridan

Mathew Shorstein

Lisa Silverman

Helen Sims-Williams

Caleigh Sinclair

Anita Singh

Vicky Singleton

Hannah Skelton

Liz Skinner

Nicola Slater-Arnold

Nicola Slawson

Olivia Smales

Sue Smallidge

Alice Smith

Beck Smith

Amanda Smith

Katharina Smith-Muller

Milly Smythe

Teny Soglia

Barbara Speed

Victoria Spring

Ella St John McGrand

Caroline Stafford

Michelle Stainer

Hannah Stark

Eleanor Steafel

Milou Stella

Catherine Stephenson

Katrina Stevens

Nina Stibbe

Jocelyn Stirling

Helen Stokes

Daniella Graham Stollery

Cat Strawbridge

Taryn Strong

Ruth Sutherland

Cass Swift

Lizzie Tait

Laura Tannenbaum

Josephine Tapper

Ruth Taylor

Helen Taylor

Katie Taylor

Melissa Taylor

Jennifer Taylor

Jess Tennant

Kate Tetlow

Debby Thomas

Hannah Thomas

Alice Thomas

Joni Thompson

Kate Tilbury

Grace Timothy

Sylvia Timothy
Joanna Tindall
Carla Tiramani Dayes
Mike Tobyn
Sonja Todd
Francesca Treadaway
Helen Trenchard
Alice Turner
Karen Tuzman
Alice Tyler
William Tyler
Leanne Tyreman-Guest
Sophia Ufton
Karen Unger
Stefanie V.
Tom Valentine
Joanna Valentine
Sara Vali
Diana Van der Lely
Kiran Vara Rawlings
Hannah Vaughan Jones
Gemma Vayro
Vanessa Veiock
Thom Venables-Gordon
Laura Vico
Sally Victoria
Vanessa Villanueva
Alice Vincent
Jessica Voge
Alice von Simson
Claire Wainwright

Sarah Wallace
Sara-Jane Wallbridge
Clementine Wallop
Katy Ward
Sarah Ward
Miranda Ward
Alexandra Watson
Amy Wearne
Jenny Wearne
Nigel Wearne
Helen Webster
Julie Wellock
Amy Westwick
Jan Westwick
Laura Whateley
Katherine Wheatley
Julie Wheeler
Tamzin Whelan
Sarah Whitby
Terri White
Phip Whitehead
Charlotte Whitfield
Allegra Whittaker
Alice Wickham
Lily Wiggins
Harriet Wileman
Megan Wiley
Diana Wilkinson
Ffion Williams
Clare Williams
James Conrad Williams

Hannah C Williams
Kelly and Jon Williams
"Welsh Kate" Williams
Danielle Willox-Semple
Sophie Wilson
Linda Wintle
H Wood
Ruth Wood
Oli Wood
Susanna Woodcock

Lou Woodhouse
Alix Wooding
Hanna Woodside
Michelle Woolfenden
Sarah Woolhouse
Ellie Wright
Julia Young Nutrition
Helen Zaltzman
Helga Zuccaro
Charlie Zygmunt